8-11-94

Highlights Of Ancient Acupuncture Prescriptions

HIGHLIGHTS

OF ANCIENT ACUPUNCTURE PRESCRIPTIONS

TRANSLATED BY
HONORA LEE WOLFE
AND
ROSE CRESCENZ

BLUE POPPY PRESS

Published by:

BLUE POPPY PRESS
1775 LINDEN AVE.
BOULDER, CO 80304

FIRST EDITION
MAY 1991

ISBN 0-936185-23-6
Library of Congress Catalog # 91-072617

Printed at Westview Press, Boulder, CO

This book is printed on archive quality, acid free, recycled paper.

Foreword

This small volume began as a class translation project in 1987 when Rose Crescenz and myself were still in acupuncture school. It was a long project and was not finished at that time. Nonetheless, there were two other people in the class, Lars Cordova and Steven Hollifield, who participated in the initial work on this translation and whom we would like to thank for their contribution. Additionally, Zhang Ting-liang, who was our translation class instructor, was very helpful with clarifying difficult passages at different points during the completion of this work. Finally we would like to acknowledge Bob Flaws, who spent many hours with us refining the terminology so that it would be as close as possible to the Chinese version.

As reference materials we used many texts and articles, but when questions arose our major source for terminology was *A Glossary of Chinese Medical Terminology and Acupuncture Points* by Nigel Wiseman, Paradigm Publications. While I personally often find the words he chooses to be somewhat unwieldy, they are technically accurate and not tainted with the confusion that is often true with some of the terminology used in prior English language translations. For standard meridian point numbers, we have chosen to use the numbering system in *Essentials of Chinese Acupuncture*, Foreign Language Press. We found, however, that *Acupuncture, A Comprehensive Text*, Bensky and O'Connor, Eastland Press, had a better selection of extra points and where possible we have listed the numbers from that text for those points. However, since all the sources for the material translated here are over 100 years old, many extra point names were not listed in available modern texts and therefore have no modern point number.

It is our hope in translating this work that it will be useful to a broad spectrum of practitioners in relieving their patients' ills.

Honora Lee Wolfe
May, 1991

Preface

Highlights of Ancient Acupuncture Prescriptions is based on Liao Run-long's Qing Dynasty *Zhen Jiu Ji Cheng (A Compilation of Acupuncture & Moxibustion)*. This is a collection of empirically proven, ancient and moxibustion formulas abstracted by Liao from Jin, Yuan, Ming, and Qing Dynasty classics of this art. Blue Poppy Press has chosen to publish this translation by Honora Lee Wolfe and Rose Crescenz for two reasons.

First, this book is an example of a pre-TCM style of Chinese acupuncture. Traditional Chinese Medicine (TCM) is the official, standardized style of Chinese medicine in the People's Republic of China. This is an herbalized style of Chinese medicine based on diagnosis by *bian zheng* or the discrimination of patterns of disharmony. However, the application of this diagnostic methodology to the formulation of acupuncture treatments is a recent addition to the practice of acupuncture. Up until the middle of present century, acupuncture formulas recorded in the literature were categorized by *bian bing* and not *bian zheng*. *Bian bing* means discrimination of disease. Prior to the 1950's acupuncture formulas were arranged according to the Chinese disease categories. This book is a collection of pre-TCM acupuncture formulas arranged according the *bian bing*. As such, it is a good example of how Chinese acupuncturists recorded their most successful treatments up until so-called liberation.

Secondly, this book is a compilation of time-tested, efficacious formulas for the beginning practitioner. Leaving aside the question of whether the TCM methodology of composing acupuncture formulas is the best and most organic methodology for this art, few beginning practitioners can do an accurate, individualized *bian zheng* diagnosis. Therefore, few beginning acupuncturists can compose accurate, individualized acupuncture treatments by this method. As a teacher of TCM, I have seen this cause a great deal of frustration and confusion among Western neophytes who cannot make this system work for them.

It is my belief and experience that the TCM methodology should be reserved for internists or specialists in what it calls *nei ke*. *Nei ke* or internal medicine implies the internal administration of medicine. TCM *bian zheng* diagnosis and the composition of polypharmacy prescription based on such diagnosis is a great methodology for practicing internal medicine. However, internal medicine should be a post-graduate study and should not be taught to beginners. Such *bian zheng* diagnosis is a highly rational process requiring more than usual logical and conceptual skills. It is not easy to master even by Chinese.[1] It is almost impossible to master *except in Chinese*. Therefore, I believe training in this methodology should be reserved for those with the knowledge, experience, and intelligence capable of mastering this approach. This is not the rank and file of current American acupuncture students.

My original acupuncture teacher, Dr. (Eric) Tao Xi-yu was of the opinion that beginners should primarily focus on learning and employing acupuncture formulas based on a *bian bing* or disease discrimination diagnosis. Although practitioners employing such empirical formulas may not cure every patient (since a single disease may be due to different patterns in different patients), still, if the formulas are good ones, they will benefit the majority of patients with a given disease or symptom. Beginners need something simple and straight forward in which to put their faith. Confidence, which is related to intention, is an extremely important component of any medical treatment. Because of the close connection between *qi* and *yi* or mind, confidence may play an especially important role in the practice of acupuncture which is the direct manipulation of *qi*.

Over the last 10 years I have known and met scores of acupuncturists both Oriental and American. Of these there has been a wide range in intelligence and education. But one thing I have noticed is that clinical efficacy rests more on faith in one's methodology than on the brilliance or sophistication of one's concepts about that methodology. In my experience, most recent graduates of American acupuncture schools are confused. They cannot do TCM *bian zheng* diagnosis accurately and with confidence. They have been exposed in an eclectic way to a number of different methodologies - Chinese, English, Japanese, Korean, and French - and typically lack a strong, central core of belief and practice. In my opinion, they have been exposed to too much too soon.

It was Dr. Tao's opinion that it takes years to learn how to do an individualized diagnosis and to compose effective acupuncture treatment based on such diagnosis. Certainly this is my experience. After several years of frustration trying to teach TCM methodology to beginners I realized that I was asking students to develop in a way and at a pace I never had myself. That such compendia of formulas lend themselves to "cookbook acupuncture" is not necessarily a criticism. Beginning cooks need cookbooks until they have gained enough experience to alter and create recipes on their own. In the same way, I see nothing wrong with beginning acupuncturists relying on empirical formulas. Hopefully, after gaining experience and the insight that goes with experience, practitioners will begin to see the rationale behind such formulas. At that point, they then can modify such formulas and compose others by themselves.

However, until that insight dawns, compendia of such formulas as contained herein do serve an important and useful function.

Bob Flaws
May, 1991

CONTENTS

FOREWORD

iii

PREFACE

v

INTERNAL CONDITIONS

1

1) *Jing* (Essence)   1
2) *Qi* (Qi)   2
3) *Shen* (Spirit)   3
4) *Xue* (Blood)   5
5) *Meng* (Dreams)   6
6) *Sheng Yin* (Voice)   7
7) *Yan Yu* (Speech)   7
8) *Jin Ye* (Body Fluids)   8
9) *Tan Yin* (Phlegm Fluid)   9
10) *Bao Gong* (Uterus)   9
11) *Chong* (Parasites)   11
12) *Xiao Bian* (Urination)   11
13) *Da Bian* (Defecation)   13

EXTERNAL CONDITIONS

15

1) *Tou* (Head)   15
2) *Nian* (Face)   17
3) *Mu* (Eye)   17
4) *Er* (Ear)   20

5) *Bi* (Nose)   21
6) *Kou* (Mouth)   22
7) *She* (Tongue)   23
8) *Ya* (Teeth)   24
9) *Yan Hou*
      (Pharynx/Larynx
      [Throat])   24
10) *Jiang Xiang*
      (Neck/Back of Neck) 26
11) *Bei* (Upper Back)   26
12) *Xiong* (Chest)   27
13) *Xie* (Flank/Intercostal
      Region)   30
14) *Ru* (Breast)   31
15) *Fu* (Abdomen)   32
16) *Yao* (Low Back)   33
17) *Shou* (Hand/Upper
      Limb)   34
18) *Zu* (Foot/Lower
      Limb)   36
19) *Pi* (Skin)   40
20) *Rou* (Flesh)   40
21) *Mai* (Vessels)   40
22) *Jin* (Sinews)   41
23) *Gu* (Bones)   42
24) *Qian Yin* (Front Yin
      i.e., Genitalia)   42
25) *Hou Yin* (Back Yin
      i.e. Anus)   47

MISCELLANEOUS CONDITIONS
49

1) *Feng* (Wind)   49
2) *Han* (Cold)   51

3) *Shi* (Damp) 56

4) *Huo* (Fire) 56

5) *Nei Shang* (Internal
  Injury) 57

6) *Xu Lao* (Empty
  Taxation) 59

7) *Ke Chuan* (Cough and
  Wheezing) 59

8) *Ou Tu* (Vomiting) 61

9) *Zhang Man* (Distention
  and Fullness) 62

10) *Fu Zhong* (Superficial
  Edema) 64

11) *Ji Ju* (Accumulations
  and Lumps) 65

12) *Huang Dan*
  (Jaundice) 66

13) *Nue Ji* (Malarial
  Disease) 67

14) *Wen Yi* (Pestilential
  or Acute Communicable
  Disease) 69

15) *Dian Xian* (Epilepsy) 70

16) *Fu Ren* (Women i.e.,
  Gynecology) 73

17) *Xiao Er* (Children i.e.,
  Pediatrics) 75

18) *Yang Zhong* (Ulcerous
  Sores and Swellings)76

Index 79

1

Internal Conditions

1) *JING* (Essence)

(1) **Wet dreams; spermatorrhea:** Either needle or moxa *Gao Huang Shu* (Bl 43), *Shen Shu* (Bl 23), *Zhong Ji* (CV 3), *Guan Yuan* (CV 4), and *Bai Huan Shu* (Bl 30). One *luo* from the foot *tai yang* bladder channel circulates from this point (Bl 30) around the front of the spinal column at the level of the waist, then returns to its main channel at Bl 31. Another name for this point is white turbidity (*Bai Zhou*) because it can be used to treat *bai dai* or white, turbid leukorrhea.

(2) **Spermatorrhea without dreams:** Moxa *Shen Shu* (Bl 23), *Guan Yuan* (CV 4), and *Zhong Ji* (CV 3).

(3) **Overflow of essence; essence full to the brim:** Needle *Zhong Ji* (CV 3), *Da He* (Ki 12) which is a confluential point of the kidney channel and the *Chong Mai, Ran Gu* (Ki 2), and *Tai Chong* (Liv 3).

(4) **Turbid essence spontaneously flows:** Moxa *Zhong Ji* (CV 3), *Guan Yuan* (CV 4), *Zu San Li* (St. 36), *Shen Shu* (Bl 23).

(5) **Empty fatigue leads to loss of essence:** Moxa *Da He* (Ki 12), and *Zhong Feng* (Liv 4).

(6) **Loss of sperm due to the five organs being empty and exhausted:** Moxa *Qu Gu* (CV 2), 40 cones on this one point, which is located at the middle of the bone above the male genitalia.

2) *Qi* (Qi)

(1) **Every kind of disorder of the qi:** One must either needle or moxa *Qi Hai* (CV 6).

(2) **Inverted qi:** Needle *Chi Ze* (Lu 5), *Shang Qiu* (Sp 5), *Tai Bai* (Sp 3), *San Yin Jiao* (Sp 6).

(3) **Sighing with upward inversion of qi:** Needle *Tai Yuan* (Lu 9) and *Shen Men* (Ht 7).

(4) **Shortness of breath:** For people with full qi needle *Da Ling* (Per 7) and *Chi Ze* (Lu 5). For those with empty qi moxa *Da Zhui* (GV 14), *Fei Shu* (Bl 13), *Shen Que* (CV 8), *Gan Shu* (Bl 18), and *Yu Ji* (Lu 10).

(5) **Diminished qi:** Either needle or moxa *Jian Shi* (Per 5), *Shen Men* (Ht 7), *Da Ling* (per 7), *Shao Chong* (Ht 9), *Zu San Li* (St 36), *Xia Lian* (LI 8), *Xing Jian* (Liv 2), *Ran Gu* (Ki 2).

(6) **Rising qi:** Moxa *Tai Chong* (Liv 3).

(7) **Lack of qi, i.e. yawning:** Needle *Tong Li* (Ht 5) and *Nei Ting* (St 44).

(8) **Qi knotted; food not dispersed:** *Tai Chang* (Supreme Granary) is another name for *Zhong Wan* (CV 12).

(9) **Pain due to chilly qi below the navel:** Moxa 100 cones on *Guan Yuan* (CV 4).

(10) **Chaotic qi of the heart:** Choose *Shen Men* (Ht 7) and *Da Ling* (Per 7).

(11) **Chaotic qi of the lung:** Choose *Yu Ji* (LI 10) and *Tai Xi* (Ki 3).

(12) **Chaotic qi of the intestine/stomach:** Choose *Tai Bai* (Sp 3), *Xian Gu* (St 43), and *Zu San Li* (St 36).

(13) **Chaotic qi of the head:** Choose *Tian Zhu* (Bl 10), *Da Shu* (Bl 11), *Tong Gu* (Bl 66), and *Shu Gu* (Bl 65).

(14) **Chaotic qi in the arm or leg:** Choose *Er Jian* (LI 2), *San Jian* (LI 3), *Nei Ting* (St 44), *Xian Gu* (St 43), *Ye Men* (TH 2), *Zhong Zhu* (Th 3), *Xia Xi* (GB 43), *Zu Ling Qi* (GB 41).

3) *SHEN* (Spirit)

(1) **Essence spirit withered:** Moxa *Guan Yuan* (CV 4) and *Gao Huang Shu* (Bl 43).

(2) **Tendency to fear; heart wary:** Needle or moxa *Ran Gu* (Ki 2), *Nei Guan* (Per 6), *Yin Ling Quan* (Sp 9), *Xia Xi* (GB 43), and *Xing Jian* (Liv 2).

(3) **Heart dread; big pounding**: Needle *Da Ling* (Per 7) and *Zu San Li* (St 36).

Comment: *Xin Xia Dan Dan* is another Chinese way of describing this condition - Wiseman translates this as a rolling

3

sensation below the heart. See *Glossary of Chinese Medical Terms and Acupuncture Points* page 314.

(4) **Impaired memory:** Needle or moxa (Lu 7), *Xin Shu* (B1 15), *Shen Men* (Ht 7), *Zhong Wan* (CV 12), *Zu San Li* (St 36), *Shao Hai* (Ht 3), and *Bai Hui* (GV 20).

(5) **Lack of will; dullness and stupidity:** Moxa *Shen Men* (Ht 7), *Zhong Chong* (Per 9), *Gui Yuen* (extra point on the back of the hand; one of the 18 ghost points; exact location unknown); *Jiu Wei* (CV 15), *Bai Hui* (GV 20), *Hou Xi* (SI 3), *Da Zhong* (Ki 4).

(6) **Hysteric raving and laughter:** Needle *Shen Men* (Ht 7), *Nei Guan* (Per 6), *Jui Wei* (CV 15), and *Feng Long* (St 40).

(7) **Epilepsy:** If the onset of the fit is at night, treat the *Yang Qiao Mai* point *Shen Mai* (B1 62); if it develops in the day use the *Yin Qiao Mai* point *Zhao Hai* (Ki 6). Moxa respectively 14 cones. Then moxa *Bai Hui* (GV 20) and *Feng Chih* (GB 20).

(8) **Manic disease:** Choose *Jiu Wei* (CV 15), *Hou Xi* (SI 3), *Yong Quan* (Ki 1), *Xin Shu* (B1 15), *Yang Jiao* (GB 33), *San Li* (St 36), *Tai Chong* (Liv 3), *Jian Shi* (Per 5), *Shang Wan* (CV 13).

(9) **Violent mania:** Choose *Feng Long* (St 40), *Ju Que* (CV 14), *Wen Liu* (LI 7), *Tong Gu* (B1 66), *Zhu Bin* (Ki 9), *Hou Xi* (SI 3), *Yin Gu* (Ki 10). Additionally moxa 30 cones on *Jian Shi* (Per 5) or 100 cones on *Tian Shu* (St 25).

4) *XUE* (Blood)

(1) **Nose bleed, vomiting blood, any loss of blood from the lower part of the body:** Needle *Yin Bai* (Sp 1), *Da Ling* (Per 7), *Shen Men* (Ht 7), and *Tai Xi* (Ki 3).

(2) **Ceaseless nose bleed:** Moxa *Xin Men* (same as *Xin Hui* [GV 22]), *Shang Xing* (GV 23), *Da Zhui* (GV 14), or use a prismatic needle to bleed *Qi Chong* (St 30), then needle *He Gu* (LI 4), *Nei Ting* (St 44), *Zu San Li* (St 36), and *Zhao Hai* (Ki 6).

(3) **Vomiting blood:** Needle *Feng Fu* (GV 16), *Da Zhui* (GV 14), *Shan Zhong* (CV 17), *Shang Wan* (CV 13), *Zhong Wan* (CV 12), *Qi Hai* (CV 6), *Guan Yuan* (CV 4), *Zu San Li* (St 36), or moxa *Da Ling* (Per 7).

(4) **Vomiting:** Needle *Shang Wan* (CV 13), *Da Ling* (Per 7), *Xi Men* (Per 4), *Shen Men* (Ht 7), and *Yu Ji* (Lu 10).

Comment: Although this literally says vomiting, we take this to be hemoptysis or coughing up blood due to the use of *Yu Ji* (Lu 10), the fire point of the lung channel which is indicated for hemoptysis.

(5) **Blood in the feces:** (If the) *guan* pulse (position) is hollow, profuse blood will come out with the feces. (In that case) moxa *Ge Shu* (Bl 17).

(6) **Coughing blood:** Needle *Lie Que* (Lu 7), *Zu San Li* (St 36), *Bai Lao* (extra point), *Fei Shu* (Bl 13), *Ru Gen* (St 18), and *Feng Men* (Bl 12).

(7) **Vomiting blood due to emptiness and taxation:** Moxa

5

Zhong Wan (CV 12), *Fei Shu* (B1 13), and *Zu San Li* (St 36).

(8) Ceaseless bleeding from the mouth and/or nose: Moxa 50 cones on *Shang Xing* (GV 23).

(9) Ceaseless bleeding from the lower part of the body: Moxa seven cones on the vertebral process just opposite of the navel (the 14th vertebrae).

Comment: This point is just above *Ming Men* (GV 4) right over the top of the vertebral process.

5) *MENG* (Dreams)

(1) Fright palpitations, insomnia: Needle *Yin Jiao* (CV 7).

(2) Vexation; unable to lie down: Needle *Yin Xi* (Ht 6).

(3) Heaviness; sleepiness: sleeping too much: Moxa one cone on the dorsal side of the most proximal joint of the ring finger. Find the point when the fingers are bent.

(4) Terrified; unable to lie down to sleep: Needle or moxa *Qiao Yin* (GB 11).

Comment: The Chinese term used here for terrified is literally *dan han* or "cold gallbladder", relating the gallbladder to timidity/courage and thus explaining the choice of the point treated.

(5) Too many dreams; tendency to be easily startled: Needle *Shen Men* (Ht 7), *Xin Shu* (B1 15), *Nei Ting* (St 44).

6) *SHENG YIN* (Voice)

(1) **Sudden muteness with asthma:** Choose (neck) *Fu-tu* (LI 18) and *Lian Quan* (CV 23).

(2) **Suddenly unable to make a sound:** Needle *Tian Tu* (CV 22).

(3) **Inverted qi: throat not capable of speaking:** Needle *Zhao Hai* (Ki 6).

Comment: Inverted qi in this context implies loss of consciousness.

(4) **Throat obstruction leading to muteness:** Needle *Feng Long* (St 40).

(5) **Sudden muteness:** Needle *He Gu* (LI 4), *Yang Jiao* (GB 35), *Tong Gu* (Ki 20), *Tian Ding* (LI 17), *Qi Men* (Liv 14), *Zhi Gou* (TH 6), and *Yong Quan* (Ki 1).

Comment: There are two points named *Tong Gu*, Ki 20 and Bl 66. Ki 20 is specific for muteness.

7) *YAN YU* (Speech)

(1) **Sudden (unexpected) loss of voice:** Choose *Shen Men* (Ht 7), *Yong Quan* (Ki 1).

(2) **Mute, cannot speak:** Needle *He Gu* (LI 4), *Yong Quan* (Ki 1), *Yang Jiao* (GB 35), *Tong Gu* (Ki 20), *Tian Ding* (LI 17), *Da Zhui* (GV 14), *Zhi Gou* (TH 6).

7

(3) **Stiff tongue; difficult to speak:** Needle *Tong Li* (Ht 5).

(4) **Flaccid tongue; unable to speak:** Needle *Ya Men* (GV 15).

(5) **Sublingual swelling; unable to speak:** Needle *Lian Quan* (CV 23).

8) *JIN YE* (Body Fluids)

(1) **Too much sweating:** First disperse *He Gu* (LI 4), second tonify *Fu Liu* (Ki 7).

(2) **Too little sweating:** First tonify *He Gu* (LI 4), second disperse *Fu Liu* (Ki 7).

(3) **Thief (night) sweating:** Needle *Yin Xi* (Ht 6), *Wu Li* (LI 13), *Jian Shi* (Per 5), *Zhong Ji* (CV 3), *Qi Hai* (CV 6).

(4) **Incessant thief (night) sweating:** Disperse *Yin Xi* (Ht 6).

(5) **Thief (night) sweating due to emptiness and detriment:** Needle *Bai Lao* (M-HN-30, 2 *cun* above and one *cun* lateral to *Da Zhui* [GV 14]) and *Fei Shu* (Bl 13).

Comment: Wiseman uses detriment to translate the word *sun*. (See page 260 of *Glossary*). This is an unweildy translation but is technically accurate and doesn't infringe upon the translation of other Chinese terms.

(6) **Cold injury; sweat can't come out:** Needle with dispersion *He Gu* (LI 4) and *Fu Liu* (Ki 7).

9) *TAN YIN* (Phlegm Fluid)

(1) **Phlegm fluid:** For all ordinary types of lodged phlegm, choose *Feng Long* (St 40) and *Zhong Wan* (CV 12).

(2) **Phlegm fluid in the chest with vomiting inversion; cannot eat:** Needle *Ju Que* (CV 14) and *Zu San Li* (St 36).

(3) **Overflowing phlegm:** Moxa *Zhong Wan* (CV 12).

(4) **Long term phlegm fluid with inability to recovery:** Moxa on *Gao Huang Shu* (Bl 43) will facilitate excellent healing.

(5) **The three burners jammed by water, qi charges, cannot eat:** Choose *Wei Dao* (GB 28), *Wei Shu* (St 21), and *Shen Shu* (Bl 23).

Comment: The three burners become stopped up by water. Qi then accumulates and rebels upward. The stomach cannot receive food. The condition can be associated with edema, ascites, and vomiting. For a discussion of this scenario see Sung Baek's *Classical Moxibustion in Clinical Practice*, p. 41-42, Blue Poppy Press, 1990.

10) *BAO GONG* (Uterus)

(1) **Menstruation (literally: moon flow) not adjusted, i.e. irregular menstruation:** (Choose) *Zhong Ji* (CV 3), *San Yin Jiao* (Sp 6), *Shen Shu* (Bl 23), and *Qi Hai* (CV 6).

Comment: Irregular menstruation is also called *yue jing qian hou wu ding qi*, which means menstruation ahead, behind, or at no fixed time.

9

(2) **Menstruation cut off and used up:** Needle *Zhong Ji* (CV 3), *San Yin Jiao* (Sp 6), *Shen Shu* (B1 23), *Qi Hai* (CV 6).

Comment: The term used here, *jing duan*, means menopause. The implication here is premature menopause.

(3) **Ceaseless uterine bleeding:** *Xue Hai* (Sp 10), *Yin Gu* (Ki 10), *San Yin Jiao* (Sp 6), *Xing Jian* (Liv 2), *Tai Chong* (Liv 3), *Zhong Ji* (CV 3), needle and moxa these.

Comment: The term *beng lou* literally means flood and leaking.

(4) **Red (and) white abnormal vaginal discharge:** Needle and moxa *Zhong Ji* (CV 3), *Shen Shu* (B1 23), *Qi Hai* (CV 6), *San Yin Jiao* (Sp 6), *Zhang Men* (Liv 13), *Xing Jian* (Liv 2).

(5) **Red abnormal vaginal discharge:** Needle *Zhong Ji* (CV 3), *Qi Hai* (CV 6), *Wei Zhong* (B1 40).

(6) **Red and white abnormal vaginal discharge:** Moxa *Dai Mai Xue* (GB 26).

(7) **Cui family four flowers:** The four flowers points are *Ge Shu* (B1 17) and *Dan Shu* (B1 19) and treat leukorrhea like magic.

Comment: This is an empirical treatment from the Cui family lineage for *dai xia* (vaginal discharge).

(8) **Cessation of menstruation for a long time: sudden great flooding downward:** Choose *Feng Long* (St 40), *Shi Men* (CV 5), *Qi Hai* (CV 6), *Tian Shu* (St 25), *Zhong Wan* (CV 12).

Comment: This refers to heavy menorrhagia some time after menopause mixed with profuse vaginal discharge which is a dangerous condition potentially associated with cervical or uterine cancer.

(9) **White vaginal discharge:** Needle and moxa *Qu Gu* (CV 2), *Zhi Yin* (Bl 67), *Zhong Ji* (CV 3).

11) *CHONG* (Parasites)

(1) **Exhaustion (due to parasites) (biliary ascariasis):** Moxa *Gao Huang Shu* (Bl 43), *Gui Yan* (ghost eyes, another name for Sp 1 used with Lu 11, see page 75, #2), *Si Hua Xue* (Bl 17 with Bl 19).

12) *XIAO BIAN* (Urination)

(1) **Retention of urine:** Needle *Zhao Hai* (Ki 6), *Da Dun* (Liv 1), *Wei Yang* (Bl 39), *Da Zhong* (Ki 4), *Xing Jian* (Liv 2), *Wei Zhong* (Bl 40), *Yin Ling Quan* (Sp 9), *Shi Men* (CV 5).

(2) **Urination dribbling and obstructed:** Needle *Guan Yuan* (CV 4), *San Yin Jiao* (Sp 6), *Yin Gu* (Ki 10), *Yin Ling Quan* (Sp 9), *Qi Hai* (CV 6), *Tai Xi* (Ki 3).

(3) **Stone *lin*:** Needle *Guan Yuan* (CV 4), *Qi Hai* (CV 6), *Da Dun* (Liv 1).

(4) **Qi *lin*:** (same as #3, delete *Da Dun* [Liv 1]).

(5) **Blood *lin*:** Needle *Yin Ling Quan* (Sp 10), *Guan Yuan* (CV 4), *Qi Chong* (St 30).

Comment: *Lin* is a category of disease where there is

11

dribbling, hesitancy, and difficulty urinating. Wiseman translates this as strangury.

(6) **Frequent slippery urination:** Moxa *Zhong Ji* (CV 3), Needle *Shen Shu* (B1 23), *Yin Ling Quan* (Sp 9), *Qi Hai* (CV 6), *Yin Gu* (Ki 10), *San Yin Jiao* (Sp 6).

(7) **Unrestrained enuresis:** Needle and moxa *Yin Ling Quan* (Sp 9), *Yang Ling Quan* (GB 34), *Da Dun* (Liv 1), *Qu Gu* (CV 2).

(8) **Pain in the penis:** Moxa *Xing Jian* (Liv 2), Needle *Zhong Ji* (CV 3), *Tai Xi* (Ki 3), *San Yin Jiao* (Sp 6), *Fu Liu* (Ki 7).

(9) **White turbid (urine):** Moxa *Shen Shu*: Needle *Zhang Men* (Liv 13), *Qu Quan* (Liv 8), *Guan Yuan* (CV 4), *San Yin Jiao* (Sp 6).

Comment: *Bai Zhuo* is a disease category in Chinese medicine, Refer to Bob Flaws' *Fire in the Valley: Vaginitis, Cervicitis, and Leukorrhea and Traditional Chinese Medicine*, Blue Poppy Press, June 1991, for a complete discussion. This basically describes a turbid discharge with urination.

(10) **Pain of the urethra (in women):** Needle and moxa *Yin Ling Quan* (Sp 9).

(11) **Pregnant woman cannot pass urine due to the pressure of the fetus:** Needle and moxa *Qu Gu* (CV 2), *Guan Yuan* (CV 4).

(12) **Block and repulsion counterflow retching; urination not free flowing:** First moxa *Qi Hai* (CV 6) and *Tian Shu* (St 25) each 21 cones.

Comment: This rather opaque terminology is exactly what is said in Chinese. The implication is explosive vomiting.

13) *DA BIAN* (Defecation)

(1) **Loose stools with thirst:** Moxa *Da Zhui* (GV 14) 3 to 5 cones.

(2) **Longterm diarrhea without recovery:** Moxa *Bai Hui* (GV 20) 5 to 7 cones.

(3) **Longstanding diarrhea:** Moxa *Qi Hai* (CV 6) and *Tian Shu* (St 25).

(4) **Ceaseless diarrhea:** Moxa 10 cones on *Shen Que* (CV 8). Moxa *Guan Yuan* (CV 4) 30 cones.

(5) **Unformed (semiliquid) stools:** Moxa the center of the navel and *San Yin Jiao* (Sp 6). Use this (formula) often (and the stools) will become fine.

(6) **Feast diarrhea:** Moxa *Yin Ling Quan* (Sp 9), *Ju Xu* (St 37), *Shang Lian* (LI 9), *Tai Chong* (Liv 3).

Comment: The implication of this is diarrhea due to overeating of greasy, sweet, rich food, alcohol, and other things that one might eat at a feast.

(7) **Watery diarrhea, limbs cold, pulse exhausted, belly painful, qi insufficient:** Moxa *Qi Hai* (CV 6) 100 cones.

(8) **Dysentery with blood and pus, stomach painful:** Use moxa on the lower *dan tian* area, *Fu Liu* (Ki 7), *Xiao Chang Shu*

(Bl 28), *Tian Shu* (St 25), and *Fu Ai* (Sp 16).

(9) **Chilly dysentery:** Moxa *Guan Yuan* (CV 4) 50 cones.

(10) **Abdominal urgency and rectal heaviness; tenesmus:** Needle *He Gu* (LI 4) and *Wai Guan* (TH 5).

(11) **Ceaseless dysentery:** Needle or moxa *He Gu* (LI 4), *Zu San Li* (St 36), *Yin Ling Quan* (Sp 9), *Zhong Wan* (CV 12), *Guan Yuan* (CV 6), *Tian Shu* (St 25), *Shen Que* (CV 8), and *Zhong Ji* (CV 3).

(12) **Any type of dysentery:** Moxa *Da Du* (Sp 2) 5 cones, and *Shang Qiu* (Sp 5), *Yin Ling Quan* (Sp 9) each 3 cones.

(13) **Stools stopped up:** Needle *Zhao Hai* (Ki 6), *Zhi Gou* (TH 6), and *Tai Bai* (Sp 3).

(14) **Stools not free flowing:** Needle *Er Jian* (LI 2), *Cheng Shan* (Bl 57), *Tai Bai* (Sp 3), *Da Zhong* (Ki 4), *Zu San Li* (St 36), *Yong Quan* (Ki 1), *Kun Lun* (Bl 60), *Zhao Hai* (Ki 6), *Zhang Men* (Liv 13), and *Qi Hai* (CV 6).

(15) **Urine and stools not free flowing in postpartum women:** Needle *Qi Hai* (CV 6), *Zu San Li* (St 36), *Guan Yuan* (CV 4), *San Yin Jiao* (Sp 6), and *Yin Gu* (Ki 10).

2

External Conditions

1) *TOU* (Head)

(1) **Dizziness/vertigo:** Needle or moxa *Shen Ting* (GV 24), *Shang Xing* (GV 23), *Xin Hui* (GV 22), *Qian Ding* GV 21), *Hou Ding* (GV 19), *Nao Kong* (GB 19), *Feng Chih* (GB 20), *Yang Gu* (SI 5), *Da Du* (Sp 2), *Zhi Yin* (B1 67), *Jin Men* (B1 63), *Shen Mai* (B1 62), *Zu San Li* (St 36). Choose appropriately from among the above points.

(2) **Dizziness and vertigo with fear of cold:** The person must wear a padded cotton hat even in Spring and Summer. If it is taken away the symptoms will recur. In this case, needle or moxa *Bai Hui* (GV 20), *Shang Xing* (GV 23), *Feng Chi* (GB 20), and *Feng Long* (St 40).

(3) **Migraine headaches:** Needle *Si Zhu Kong* (TH 23), *Feng Chi* (GB 20), *He Gu* (LI 4), *Zhong Wan* (CV 12), *Jie Xi* (St 41), and *Zu San Li* (St 36).

(4) **Regular headache:** Needle *Shang Xing* (GV 23), *Shen Ting* (GV 24), *Tai Yang* (Extra Point), and *Bai Hui* (GV 20).

Comment: A regular headache implies bilateral or ambilateral headache.

(5) **Kidney inversion headache:** Moxa 100 cones on *Guan Yuan* (CV 4).

Comment: Clear yang is not ascending above, leading to empty headache.

(6) **Counterflow inversion headache and tooth pain:** Moxa 10 cones on *Qu Bin* (GB 7).

(7) **Phlegm inversion headache:** Needle *Feng Long* (St 40).

(8) **Head wind headache:** Needle *Bai Hui* (GV 20). Moxa *Xin Hui* (GV 22), *Qian Ding* (GV 21), *Shang Xing* (GV 23), and *Bai Hui* (GV 20).

(9) **Head wind:** Needle and moxa *Shang Xing* (GV 23), *Qian Ding* (CV 21), *Bai Hui* (GV 20), *Yang Gu* (SI 5), *Guan Chong* (TH 1), *Kun Lun* (B1 60), choosing what is needed.

(10) **Headache (at the) nape (of the neck with) opisthotonis:** First reduce and then tonify *Cheng Jiang* (CV 24), then needle *Feng Fu* (GV 16).

(11) **Head wind with red face and eyes:** Needle *Tong Li* (Ht 5), and *Jie Xi* (St 41).

(12) **Head wind with dizziness:** Needle *He Gu* (LI 4), *Feng Long* (St 40), *Jie Xi* (St 41), and *Feng Chi* (GB 20).

(13) **Head and neck unyielding straight (cannot turn or bend neck):** Needle and moxa *Feng Fu* (GV 16).

(14) **Entire head and neck painful:** Needle *Bai Hui* (GV 20), *Hou Ding* (GV 19), and *He Gu* (LI 4).

(15) **Superciliary ridge pain:** Needle *Zhan Zhu* (BL 2), *He Gu* (LI 4), *Shen Ting* (GV 24), *Tou Wei* (St 8), *Jie Xi* (St 41).

(16) **Brain pain, brain chilly, brain dizziness:** Needle *Xin Hui* (GV 22).

(17) **One-sided headache becomes bilateral:** Choose the *ah-shi* points and needle them, the patient will presently recover.

(18) **Headache after intoxication:** Choose the extra point *Yin Tang, Zhan Zhu* (B1 2), *Zu San Li* (St 36), *Feng Men* (B1 12), and *Shan Zhong* (CV 17) and needle them.

2) *NIAN* (Face)

(1) **Face swollen:** Moxa *Shui Fen* (CV 9).

(2) **Face itchy (and) swollen:** Needle *Ying Xiang* (LI 20) and *He Gu* (LI 4).

(3) **Cheeks swollen:** Needle *Jia Che* (St 6) and *He Gu* (LI 4).

(4) **Face (and) eyes too swollen to move:** Mostly puncture to bleed the small blood vessel in the depression inside the elbow.

3) *MU* (Eye)

(1) **Eyeball pain:** Needle *Feng Fu* (GV 16), *Feng Chi* (GB 20), *Tong Li* (Ht 5), *He Gu* (LI 4), *Shen Mai* (Bl 62), *Zhao Hai* (Ki 6), *Da Dun* (Liv 1), and *Qiao Yin* (GB 11).

17

(2) **Eye red and swollen, slight corneal opacity, photophobia, and blurred vision with dryness:** Needle *Shang Xing* (GV 23), *Bai Hui* (GV 20), *Zan Zhu* (Bl 2), *Si Zhi Kong* (TB 23), *Jing Ming* (Bl 1), *Tong Zi Liao* (GB 1), *Tai Yang* (extra point), *He Gu* (LI 4). Bleed *Nei Ying Xiang* (extra point just medial to *Ying Xiang* [LI 20], but still lateral to the nostrils).

(3) **Sudden redness, swelling, and pain of the eye:** Needle *Jing Ming* (Bl 1), *He Gu* (LI 4); bleed *Tai Yang* (extra point); needle *Shang Xing* (GV 23), *Guang Ming* (GB 37), and *Di Wu Hui* (GB 42).

Comment: One Chinese interpreter suggests that this is a description of the western disease conjunctivitis.

(4) **All types of corneal opacity:** Bleed *Jing Ming* (Bl 1), *Si Bai* (St 2), *Tai Yang* (extra point), *Bai Hui* (GV 20), *Shang Yang* (LI 1), *Li Dui* (St 45), and *Guang Ming* (GB 37); moxa *He Gu* (LI 4), *Sun Li* (St 36), *Ming Men* (GV 4), *Guang Ming* (GB 37) and *Gan Shu* (Bl 18).

(5) **Triangular mucous flesh climbing the eyeball:** Bleed *Jing Ming* (Bl 1), *Feng Chi* (GB 20), *Qi Men* (Liv 14), and *Tai Yang* (extra point).

Comment: This is a description of ptergium.

(6) **Rotten bowstring wind:** Moxa 7 cones on *Gu Kong* (another name for *San Yang Luo* [TB 8]). Blow out the moxa and then bleed to ridge of the eyesocket along the bone in several places.

Comment: This refers to eroded, pitted eyelids which have the appearance of being bumpy, uneven, or chewed. It is usually seen on people who have been indigent and homeless for a long time, with irregular or inadequate diet.

(7) **Facing into a cold wind causes tearing:** Needle *Zu Ling Qi* (GB 41) and *He Gu* (LI 4) and moxa *Gu Kong* (TB 8) 7 cones on each side, blow the fire out with your mouth.

(8) **Clear-eyed blindness:** Moxa *Ju Liao* (St 3); needle *Ming Men* (GV 4), and *Shang Yang* (LI 1).

Comment: This condition corresponds to glaucoma in western medicine.

(9) **Eyes dim:** Moxa *San Li* (St 36); needle *Cheng Qi* (St 1), *Gan Shu* (Bl 18), and *Tong Zi Liao* (GB 1).

(10) **Night blindness:** Needle or bleed *Shen Ting* (GV 24), *Shang Xing* (GV 23), *Qian Ding* (GV 21), *Bai Hui* (GV 20), *Jing Ming* (Bl 1), then perhaps moxa *Gan Shu* (Bl 18) and *Zhao Hai* (Ki 6).

(11) **Sudden blindness; cannot see objects:** Bleed *Zan Zhu* (Bl 2), *Tai Yang* (extra point), *Shang Xing* (GV 23), and *Nei Ying Xiang* (extra point).

(12) **Pupil swollen and painful; eyeball almost coming out:** Bleed *Ba Guan* (extra point, another name for *Ba Xie*) between the fingers.

(13) **Eye rolls up and back:** Moxa each of the vertebra from C2 through C5 seven cones each. Light them simultaneously.

(14) **Eye itches and aches:** Needle *Guang Ming* (GB 37) and *Di Wu Hui* (GB 42).

(15) **Eyelashes fall (out):** Needle *Si Zhu Kong* (TB 23).

19

(16) **Cataract:** Moxa *Zu Lin Qi* (GB 41) and *Gan Shu* (Bl 18) 7 cones on each.

(17) **Cataracts with red nebula:** Needle *Tai Yuan* (Lu 9), *Xia Xi* (GB 43), *Zan Zhu* (Bl 2), and *Feng Chi* (GB 20).

(18) **Red corneal opacity:** Needle *Zan Zhu* (Bl 2), *Hou Xi* (SI 3), and *Ye Men* (TB 2).

(19) **Both eyes suddenly painful:** Needle *San Jian* (LI 3).

(20) **Above and below the eye socket black:** Needle *Chi Ze* (Lu 5) to a depth of 3 *fen*.

Comment: Dark circles around the eyes is suggested here.

4) *ER* (Ear)

(1) **Tinnitus:** Needle or moxa *Bai Hui* (GV 20), *Ting Gong* (SI 19), *Er Men* (TH 21), *Shang Guan* (GB 3), *Ye Men* (TH 3), *Zhong Zhu* (TH 3), *Yang Gu* (SI 5), *Shang Yang* (LI 1), *Shen Shu* (Bl 23), *Qian Gu* (SI 2), *Wan Gu* (SI 4), *(Tou) Lin Qi* (GB 15), *Yang Xi* (LI 5), *Pian Li* (LI 6), *He Gu* (LI 4), *Da Ling* (Per 7), *Tai Xi* (Ki 3), and *Jin Men* (Bl 63).

Comment: This group of points is obviously not intended to be a single formula but a list from which to choose depending upon which Channels seem to be most affected, or points to rotate if frequent treatments are being given.

(2) **Deafness:** Needle *Zhong Zhu* (TH 3), *Wai Guan* (TH 5), *He Liao* (LI 19), *Ting Hui* (GB 2), *Ting Gong* (SI 19), *He Gu* (LI 4), *Shang Yang* (LI 1), and *Zhong Chong* (Per 9).

20

(3) **Pus and water flows from ear:** Needle *Er Men* (TH 21), *Yi Feng* (TH 17), and *He Gu* (LI 4).

(4) **Sudden deafness:** Needle *Tian You* (TH 16), and *Si Du* (TH 9).

(5) **Hard of hearing:** Needle *Er Men* (TH 21), *Feng Chi* (GB 20), *Tai Xi* (Ki 3), *Yi Feng* (TH 17), *Ting Hui* (GB 2), and *Ting Gong* (SI 19).

(6) **Sudden deafness moxa method:** Use a piece of *Cang Zhu* (Rhizoma Atractylodes) about 7 *fen* (3/4 of an inch) long. One end should be flat and one end whittled to point into the opening of the ear like a cone. Moxa 7 cones on the flat side. If during sleep the inside of the ear becomes very hot, there will be a prompt effect.

5) *BI* (Nose)

(1) **Runny nose, clear or possibly turbid mucous:** Moxa 27 cones on *Shang Xing* (GV 23), also needle *Ren Zhong* (GV 26), *Feng Fu* (GV 16). (If) this is not effective, needle *Bai Hui* (GV 20), *Feng Chi* (GB 20), *Feng Men* (Bl 12), and *Da Zhui* (GV 14).

(2) **Nose stuffed (and) unable to distinguish fragrant from foul smells:** Needle *Ying Xiang* (LI 20), *Shang Xing* (GV 23), *He Gu* (LI 4). (If this is) not effective, moxa *Ren Zhong (GV 26), Bai Lao* (M-HN-30, located 2 *cun* above and 1 *cun* lateral to *Da Zhui* [GV 14]), *Feng Fu* (GV 16), and *Qian Gu* (SI 2).

(3) **Runny nose (with an) abominable smell:** Needle (or) moxa *Shang Xing* (GV 23), *Qu Chai* (Bl 4), *He Gu* (LI 4),

Ying Xiang (LI 20), and *Ren Zhong* (GV 26).

(4) **Copious runny nose:** Moxa *Xin Hui* (GV 22), *Qian Ding* (GV 21), and *Ying Xiang* (LI 20).

(5) **Nasal polyps:** Needle *Feng Chi* (GB 20), *Feng Fu* (GV 16), *He Liao* (TH 22), *Ying Xiang* (LI 20), and *Ren Zhong* (GV 26).

(6) **Prolonged uncontainable flow of mucous:** Moxa *Bai Hui* (GV 20).

6) *KOU* (Mouth)

(1) **Mouth sores/ulcers:** Choose from *Cheng Jiang* (CV 24), *He Gu* (LI 4), *Ren Zhong* (GV 26), *Chang Jiang* (GV 1); also bleed *Jin, Jin, Yu Ye* (extra point); also reduce *Wei Zhong* (B1 40); moxa 7 cones each on *Hou Xi* (SI 3), *Dan Shu* (B1 19), and *Xiao Chang Shu* (B1 27); possibly use *Tai Chong* (Liv 3) and *Lao Gong* (Per 8) (as well).

(2) **Mouth dry:** Needle *Chi Ze* (Lu 5), *Qu Ze* (Per 3), *Da Ling* (Per 7), *San Jian* (LI 3), *Shao Shang* (Lu 11), and *Shang Yang*
(LI 1).

(3) **Wasting and thirst (diabetic polydipsia):** Needle and/or moxa *Shui Gou* (GV 26), *Cheng Jiang* (CV 24), *Jin Jin, Yu Ye* (extra point), *Qu Chi* (LI 11), *Lao Gong* (Per 8), *Tai Chong* (Liv 3), *Xing Jian* (Liv 2), *Ran Gu* (Ki 2), *Yin Bai* (Sp 1).

(4) **Lips dry (but) saliva is present:** Needle *Xia Lian* (LI 8).

(5) **Lips dry; cannot swallow:** Needle *San Jian* (LI 3) and *Shao Shang* (Lu 11).

(6) **Lips move like worms:** Needle and/or moxa *Shui Gu* (GV 26).

Comment: This describes a feeling as if worms are crawling on the lips.

(7) **Lip swollen:** Needle *Ying Xiang* LI 20).

(8) **Mouth silent; (can) not open:** Needle and/or moxa *Jia Che* (St 6), *Shi Gou* (TH 6), *Wai Guan* (TH 5), *Lie Que* (Lu 7) and *Li Dui* (St 45).

7) *SHE* (Tongue)

(1) **Tongue swollen; hard to speak:** Use a triangular needle to bleed *Lian Quan* (CV 23), and *Jin Jin, Yu Ye* (extra point), Needle *Tian Tu* (CV 22), *Shao Shang* (Lu 11), *Ran Gu* (Ki 2), and *Feng Fu* (GV 16) in the normal fashion.

(2) **Tongue rolled up:** Needle *Ye Men* (TH 2) and *Er Jian* LI 2).

(3) **Tongue extremely swollen (like a pig's uterus):** Use a (triangular) needle to prick the large vessel below the tongue. Blood will immediately come out. Be sure not to prick the center vein, because if the bleeding doesn't stop, the patient may die. If this happens, cauterize the area with a piece of red hot copper wire, or apply a mixture of straw ashes mixed with vinegar and this will alleviate the wound. Most people are unaware of the seriousness of this condition. If not

treated properly the person may die.

(4) **Tongue stiff, saliva (drips) down:** Moxa *Yang Gu* (SI 5).

(5) **Stiff tongue:** Needle *Ya Men* (GV 15), *Shao Shang* (Lu 11), *Yu Ji* (Lu 10), *Zhong Chong* (Per 9), *Yin Gu* (Ki 10), and *Ran Gu* (Ki 2).

(6) **Flaccid tongue:** Needle *Feng Fu* (GV 16), *Tai Yuan* (Lu 9), *Nei Ting* (St 44), *He Gu* (LI 4), *Chong Yang* (St 42), and *San Yin Jiao* (Sp 6).

8) *YA* (Teeth)

(1) **Tooth pain:** Needle *He Gu* (LI 4).

(2) **Upper tooth pain:** Needle *Ren Zhong* (GV 26), *Tai Yuan* (Lu 9), *Lu Xi* (point unknown), *Zu San Li* (St 26), and *Nei Ting* (St 44).

(3) **Lower tooth pain:** Needle *Cheng Jiang* (CV 24), *He Gu* (LI 4), and *Jia Che* (St 6).

9) *YAN HOU* (Pharynx/Larynx [Throat])

(1) **Throat shut:** Needle *Shao Shang* (Lu 11), *He Gu* (LI 4), *Chi Ze* (Lu 5); also needle *Guan Chong* (TH 1), and *Qiao Yin* (GB 44 or GB 11).

Comment: The text does not specify whether one should use *Zu Qiao Yin* or *Tou Qiao Yin*. Other sources list both points for usage in constriction or blockage of the throat.

(2) **Pharynx obstructed:** Inside (there is) malign blood, (if one) pierces (a vessel), (the patient will) spontaneously recover.

(3) **(Vocal) chord (larynx) wind:** Needle *Shao Shang* (Lu 11), *He Gu* (LI 4), *Feng Fu* (GV 16), and *Shang Xing* (GV 23).

(4) **Larynx obstructed:** Needle *Shen Men* (Ht 7), *Chi Ze* (Lu 5), *Da Ling* (Per 7) and *Qian Gu* (SI 2). Also/or needle *Feng Long* (St 40), *Yong Quan* (Ki 1), *Guan Chong* (TH 1), *Shao Shang* (Lu 11), and *Yin Bai* (Sp 1).

(5) **Larynx/pharynx (throat) shut (and) stopped up:** Needle *Zhao Hai* (Ki 6), *Qu Quan* (Liv 8), and *He Gu* (LI 4).

(6) **Milky moth (acute tonsilitis):** Needle and/or bleed *Shao Shang* (Lu 11), *He Gu* (LI 4), and *Yu Ye, Jin Jin* (extra point).

(7) **Laryngeal pain:** Needle *Feng Fu* (GV 16).

(8) **Year after year (longterm) obstruction (of the) larynx:** Moxa 2-3 cones on the first knuckle of the large finger (thumb). Use the left side on a man and the right side on a woman.

(9) **Food cannot pass down the throat:** Moxa *Shan Zhong* (CV 17).

(10) **Outside of throat swollen:** Needle *Ye Men* (TH 2).

(11) **Inside (of the) throat (constricted) as if a fish bone were caught inside:** Needle *Jian Shi* (Per 5) and *San Jian* (LI 3).

(12) **Throat swollen:** Needle *Zhong Zhu* (TH 3) and *Tai Xi* (Ki 3).

10) *JING XIANG* (Neck/back of neck)

(1) **Nape of the neck unyielding (stiff):** Needle *Cheng Jiang* (CV 24) and *Feng Fu* (GV 16).

(2) **Neck stiff and painful:** Needle *Tong Tian* (B1 7), *Bai Hui* (GV 20), *Feng Chi* (GB 20), *Wan Gu* (GB 12), *Ya Men* (GV 15), and *Da Shu* (B1 11).

(3) **Neck pain:** Needle *Hou Xi* (SI 3).

(4) **A swelling in the throat (goiter, mumps, lymphadenitis, hyperthyroid, etc.):** Needle *He Gu* (LI 4) and *Qu Chi* (LI 11).

(5) **Opisthotonis:** Needle *He Gu* (LI 4), *Cheng Jiang* (CV 24), and *Feng Fu* (GV 16).

11) *BEI* (Upper Back)

(1) **Spinal column stiff and painful:** Needle *Ren Zhong* (GV 26).

(2) **Upper back ache:** Needle *Shou San Li* (LI 10) with perpendicular insertion, *Jian Yu* (LI 15), *Tian Jing* (TH 10), *Qu Chi* (LI 11), and *Yang Gu* (SI 5).

(3) **Back painful, shooting into shoulder:** Needle *Wu Shu* (GB 27), *Kun Lun* (B1 60), *Xuan Zhong* (GB 39), *Jian Jing* (GB 21), and *Jia Feng* (This name was not listed in any source that we could find. The name implies a crack or fissure in a bone in the shoulder area.)

(4) **Pain of spinal column; pain all over back:** Needle/moxa

26

on *Hun Men* (Bl 47).

(5) **Upper backache:** Needle *Gao Huang Shu* (Bl 43) and *Jian Jing* (GB 21); use perpendicular insertion.

(6) **Upper back (and) shoulder sore (and) painful:** Needle *Feng Men* (Bl 12).

Comment : The word here for sore is *suan* which literally means acid or vinegar. This refers to the sore quality arising from lactic acid build up in the muscles.

(7) **Back stiff and rigid:** Needle and/or moxa *Ren Zhong* (GV 26), *Feng Fu* (GV 16), and *Fei Shu* (Bl 13). (Note: in ancient times GV 16 was forbidden to moxa).

Comment: The characters here imply that the natural curvature of the spine is gone.

(8) **Back tension:** Needle *Jing Qu* (Lu 8).

(9) **Upper back and shoulder pulling on each other:** Needle and/or moxa *Er Jian* (LI 2), *Shang Yang* (Lu 1), *Wei Zhong* (Bl 40), and *Kun Lun* (Bl 60).

Comment: One Chinese medical informant glosses this as pain shooting back and forth between the upper back and shoulders.

12) *XIONG* (Chest)

(1) **The nine categories of heart pain:** Needle or moxa *Jian Shi* (PC 5), *Ling Dao* (Ht 4), *Gong Sun* (Sp 4), *Tai Chong* (Liv

27

3), *Zu San Li* (St 36), *Yin Ling Quan* (Sp 9).

Comment: General treatment for heart pain of unknown or complicated etiology.

(2) **Abrupt or sudden heart pain:** *Ran Gu* (Ki 2), *Shang Wan* (CV 13), *Qi Hai* (CV 6), *Yong Quan* (Ki 1), *Jian Shi* (PC 5), *Zi Gong* (TH 6), *Zu San Li* (St 36), *Da Dun* (Liv 1), *Du Yin* (an extra point located beneath the 2nd toe at the center of the most proximal joint). Needle and moxa these.

(3) **Stomach cavity pain:** Needle and moxa *Zu San Li* (St 36).

(4) **Sour breast/chest pain (heartburn):** Needle and moxa *Hun Men* (B1 37).

(5) **Pain in the heart:** Needle and moxa *Nei Guan* (PC 6).

(6) **Heart pain extending in the back:** Needle and moxa *Jing Gu* (B1 64), *Kun Lun* (B1 60); if unstoppable, again needle *Ran Gu* (Ki 2), *Wei Yang* (B1 39).

(7) **Heart obstruction pain:** Needle *Ju Que* (CV 14), *Shang Ju Xu* (St 37), *Zhong Wan* (CV 12).

(8) **Pain right on the heart:** Needle and moxa *Jing Gu* (B1 64), *Kun Lun* (B1 60); if it does not stop, again needle and moxa *Ran Gu* (Ki 2), *Da Dao* (Sp 2), *Tai Bai* (Sp 3), *Tai Xi* (Ki 3), *Xing Jian* (Liv 2), *Tai Chong* Liv 3), *Yu Ji* (Lu 10).

(9) **Worm heart pain:** Choose *Shang Wan* (CV 13), *Zhong Wan* (CV 12), *Yin Du* (Ki 19).

Comment: This character *chong* means worms, parasites, and vermin in general. The implication is heart pain due to a parasitic infection. Numbers 9 and 10 are likely 2 of the 9 types of heart pain.

(10) **Blood heart pain:** Needle and moxa *Qi Men* (Liv 14).

(11) **Cold injury binding the chest:** Needle *Zhi Gou* (TH 6), *Jian Shi* (PC 5), *Xing Jian* (Liv 2). Chest accumulation moxa method: use Semen Crotonis Tiglii (*Ba Dou*) 10 pc. Peel and grind into a powder, adding 5 grams of powdered Rhizoma Coptidis (*Huang Lian*). Mix with saliva and shape into small cakes. Fill the navel with some of this dough and put the moxa on top of this. As soon as there are sounds in the abdomen (borborygmus), the disease will be gone. The specific number of cones required is not important. After finishing the moxa, with the help of a handkerchief soaked in warm water, rub the navel gently, in order to prevent superficial lesions or ulceration.

Comment: Cold injury means invasion by external cold which causes binding of the chest.

(12) **Thoracic glomus with stuffiness:** Needle and moxa *Yong Quan* (Ki 1), *Tai Xi* (Ki 3), *Zhong Chong* (Per 9), *Da Ling* (Per 7), *Yin Bai* (Sp 1), *Tai Bai* (Sp 3), *Shao Chong* (Ht 9), *Shen Men* (Ht 7).

(13) **Pain of the sub-clavicular fossa:** Needle and moxa *Tai Yuan* (Lu 9), *Shang Yang* (LI 1), and *Zu Lin Qi* (GB 41).

(14) **Fullness (stuffiness) of the chest:** Needle and moxa *Jing Qu* (Lu 8), *Yang Xi* (LI 5), *San Jian* (LI 3), *Hou Xi* (SI 3), *Jian Shi* (Per 5), *Yang Ling Quan* (GB 34), *Zu San Li* (St 36), *Qu Quan* (Liv 8), and *Zu Lin Qi* (GB 41).

(15) **Chest obstruction:** Needle and moxa *Tai Yuan* (Lu 9).

(16) **Intercostal pain:** Needle and moxa *Tian Jing* (TH 10), *Zhi Gou* (TH 6), *Jian Shi* (Per 5), *Da Ling* (Per 7), *Zu San Li* (St 36), *Tai Bai* (Sp 3), *Qiu Xu* (GB 40), and *Yang Fu* (GB 38).

(17) **Quivering of the chest (with excitement):** Needle/moxa *Jian Shi* (Per 5).

(18) **Chest fullness with swollen bronchii:** Needle *Nei Guan* (Per 6); moxa *Ge Shu* (Bl 17).

(19) **Swollen and stuffy flanks extending to the abdomen:** Needle/moxa *Xia Lian* (LI 8), *Qiu Xu* (GB 40), *Xia Xi* (GB 43), *Shen Shu* (Bl 23).

(20) **Cold inside chest:** Moxa *Shan Zhong* (CV 17).

(21) **Heart and chest pain:** Needle/moxa *Qu Ze* (Per 3), *Nei Guan* (Per 6), and *Da Ling* (Per 7).

(22) **Any type of bitter (bad) pain in the heart, chest, abdomen, flanks, ribs, upper or lower back:** Take powdered Si Chuan pepper and mix it with vinegar to form a sort of cake. Burn moxa on top of these cakes over the sore areas. As soon as the patient feels pain (from the moxa), stop (remove the moxa).

13) *XIE* (Flank or intercostal region)

(1) **Flank pain:** Needle/moxa *Xuan Zhong* (GB 39), *Qiao Yin* (GB 44), *Wai Guan* (TH 5), *Zu San Li* (St 36), *Zhi Gou* (TH 6), *Zhang Men* (Liv 13), *Zhong Feng* (Liv 4), *Yang Ling Quan* (GB 34), *Xing Jian* (Liv 2), *Qi Men* (Liv 14), and *Yin Ling Quan* (Sp 9).

(2) **Intolerable flank pain radiating to the costal region:** Needle/moxa *Qi Men* (Liv 14), *Zhang Men* (Liv 13), *Xing Jian* (Liv 2), *Qiu Xu* (GB 40), *Yong Quan* (Ki 1), *Zhi Gou* (TH 6), and *Dan Shu* (B1 19).

(3) **Flank and chest distended, painful:** Needle/moxa *Gong Sun* (Sp 4), *Zu San Li* (St 36), *Tai Chong* (Liv 3), and *San Yin Jiao* (Sp 6).

(4) **Waist and flank pain:** Needle/moxa *Huan Tiao* (GB 30), *Zhi Yin* (B1 67), *Tai Bai* (Sp 3), and *Yang Fu* (GB 38).

(5) **Flank and rib pain:** Needle *Zhi Gou* (TH 6), *Wai Guan* (TH 5), and *Qu Chi* (LI 11).

(6) **Flank pain on both sides:** Needle and/or moxa *Qiao Yin* (GB 44), *Da Dun* (Liv 1), and *Xing Jian* (Liv 2).

(7) **Flank fullness:** Needle and/or moxa *Zhang Men* (Liv 13), *Yang Gu* (SI 5), *Wan Gu* (SI 4), *Zhi Gou* (TH 6), *Gu Shu* (B1 17), and *Shen Mai* (B1 62).

(8) **Ribs and spine pulled together:** Needle/moxa *Gan Shu* (B1 18).

14) *RU* (Breast)

(1) **Jealous milk:** Needle *Tai Yuan* (Lu 9).

Comment: The term jealous milk means hypergalactia or excessive milk production. The folk meaning is that women with an overabundance of milk would be the object of other women's jealousy.

(2) **Mastitis:** Needle *Ying Chuang* (St 16), *Ru Gen* (St 18), *Shang Ju Xu* (St 37), *Xia Lian* (LI 8), *Fu Liu* (Ki 7), *Tai Xi* (Ki 3).

(3) **Pain due to mastitis:** Needle *Zu San Li* (St 36).

(4) **Agalactia:** Moxa *San Zhong* (CV 17); needle *Shao Ze* (SI 1).

(5) **Swollen breast pain:** Needle *Zu Lin Qi* (GB 41).

15) *FU* (Abdomen)

(1) **Abdominal pain:** Needle *Nei Guan* (PC 6), *Zhi Gou* (TH 6), *Zhao Hai* (Ki 6), *Ju Que* (CV 14), *Zu San Li* (St 36).

(2) **Pain of the abdomen and navel:** Needle and moxa *Yin Ling Quan* (Sp 9), *Tai Chong* (Liv 3), *Zu San Li* (St 36), *Zhi Gou* (TH 6), *Zhong Wan* (CV 12), *Guan Yuan* (CV 4), *Tian Shu* (St 25), *Gong Sun* (Sp 4), *San Yin Jiao* (Sp 6), *Yin Gu* (Ki 10).

(3) **Lancinating pain in the abdomen:** Needle and moxa *Gong Sun* (Sp 4).

(4) **Pain at the navel with watery stools (duck stool):** Moxa navel *Shen Que* (CV 8).

(5) **Accumulation pain:** Needle and moxa *Qi Hai* (CV 6), *Zhong Wan* (CV 12), *Yin Bai* (Sp 1).

Comment: The literal meaning here is indigestion from food stagnation.

(6) **Borborygmus with diarrhea:** Moxa *Shui Fen* (CV 9), *Tian Shyu* (St 25), *Shen Que* (CV 8).

(7) **Lower abdominal pain:** Needle and moxa *Xia Lian* (LI 8), *Fu Liu* (Ki 7), *Zhong Feng* (Liv 4), *Da Dun* (Liv 1), *Guan Yuan* (CV 4), *Shen Shu* (Bl 23), etc.

(8) **Intolerable acute lower abdominal pain:** Moxa *Du Yin* (an extra point located at the center of the most proximal joint of the bottom of the second toe) 5 cones. In hernia, testicular swelling, or hernia with sudden heart pain, this point is suitable.

16) *YAO* (Low Back)

(1) **Lumbar pain:** Moxa *Shen Shu* (Bl 23).

(2) **Bent over at the waist, unable to stretch up:** Bleed *Wei Zhong* (Bl 40).

(3) **Waist unable to bend forward or backward:** Needle *Ren Zhong* (GV 26), *Huan Tiao* (GB 30), *Wei Zhong* (Bl 40).

(4) **Kidney emptiness lumbar pain:** Needle and moxa *Shen Shu* (Bl 23); needle *Wei Zhong* (Bl 40).

(5) **Lumbar pain due to sprain:** Needle *Huan Tiao* (GB 30), *Wei Zhong* (Bl 40), *Kun Lun* (Bl 60), *Chi Ze* (Lu 5), *Yang Ling Quan* (GB 34), *Xia Liao* (Bl 34).

(6) **Lumbar pain with stiffness and rigidity:** Needle *Ming Men* (GV 4), *Kun Lun* (Bl 60), *Zhi Shi* (Bl 52), *Xing Jian* (Liv 2), *Fu Liu* (Ki 7).

(7) **Lumbar pain as if sitting in water:** Moxa *Yang Fu* (GB 38).

(8) **Lumbar pain, difficult to move:** Needle *Wei Zhong* (B1 40), *Xing Jian* (Liv 2), *Feng Shi* (GB 31).

17) *SHOU* (Hand and Arm)

(1) **The five fingers rigid and spastic:** Needle and moxa *Er Jian* (LI 2), *Qian Gu* (SI 2).

(2) **Pain in the five fingers:** Needle and moxa *Yang Chi* (TH 4), *Wai Guan* (TH 5), *He Gu* (LI 4).

(3) **Both hands rigid, spastic, numb:** Moxa *Da Ling* (Per 7).

(4) **Elbow contraction with irritated and protruding tendons:** Needle *Chi Ze* (Lu 5).

(5) **Hand and forearm pain, unable to lift or move:** Needle *Chi Ze* (Lu 5), *Qu Chi* (LI 11), *Jian Yu* (LI 15), *Shou San Li* (LI 10), *Shao Hai* (Ht 3), *Tai Yuan* (Lu 9), *Yang Xi* (LI 5), *Qian Gu* (SI 2), *Ye Men* (TH 2), *He Gu* (LI 4), *Wai Guan* (TB 5), and *Wan Gu* (SI 4).

(6) **Forearms cold:** Moxa *Chi Ze* (Lu 5) and *Shen Men* (Ht 7).

(7) **Inner part of the forearm cold:** Needle *Tai Yuan* (Lu 9).

(8) **Side of forearm and wrist painful:** Needle *Yang Gu* (SI 5).

(9) **Shaking of the hand and wrist:** Needle and/or moxa *Qu Ze* (Per 3).

(10) **Hands and wrists without strength:** Needle and moxa *Lie Que* (Lu 7).

(11) **Elbow, forearm, hand, and fingers cannot bend:** Needle and/or moxa *Qu Chi* (LI 11), *Shou San Li* (LI 10), *Wai Guan* (TH 5), and *Zhong Zhu* (TH 3).

(12) **Chilly pain of the hand and forearm:** Moxa *Jian Jing* (GB 21), *Qu Chi* (LI 11), and *Xia Lian* (LI 8).

(13) **Numbness of the hand and forearm:** Needle and moxa *Tian Jing* (TH 10), *Qu Chih* (LI 11), *Wai Guan* (TH 5), *Jing Qu* (Lu 8), *Zhi Gou* (TH 6), *Yang Xi* (LI 5), *Wan Gu* (SI 4), *Shang Lian* (LI 9), and *He Gu* (LI 4).

(14) **Hand and fingers rigid and tense:** Needle and moxa *Qu Chi* (LI 11), *He Gu* (LI 4), and *Yang Gu* (SI 5).

(15) **Heat in the heart of the hand:** Needle *Lao Gong* (Per 8), *Qu Chih* (LI 11), *Qu Ze* (Per 3), *Nei Guan* (Per 6), *Lie Que* (Lu 7), *Jing Qu* (Lu 8), *Tai Yuan* (Lu 9), *Zhong Chong* (Per 9), and *Shao Chong* (Ht 9).

Comment: Heart of the hand means center of the palms.

(16) **Hand and forearm red and swollen:** Needle *Qu Chi* (LI 11), *Tong Li* (Ht 5), *Zhong Zhu* (TH 3), *He Gu* (LI 4), *Shou San Li* (LI 10), and *Ye Men* (TH 2).

(17) **Heat in the center of the palms:** Needle *Lie Que* (Lu 7), *Jing Qu* (Lu 8), *Tai Yuan* (Lu 9), and *Lao Gong* (Per 8).

(18) **Inability to lift or move the shoulder and forearm:** Needle and moxa *Qu Chi* (LI 11), *Jian Yu* (LI 15), *Ju Gu* (LI 16), *Qing Leng Yuan* (TH 11), *Guan Chong* (TH 1).

(19) **Swelling of the axilla:** Needle *Chi Zi* (Lu 5), *Xiao Hai* (SI 8), *Jian Shi* (Per 5), and *Da Ling* (Per 7).

(20) **Subaxillary swelling:** Choose *Yang Fu* (GB 38), *Qiu Xu* (GB 40), *Zu Lin Qi* (GB 41).

(21) **Shoulder and forearm vexatious pain:** Needle *Jian Yu* (LI 15), *Jian Jing* (GB 21), and *Qu Chi* (LI 11).

(22) **Forearm sore and contracted:** Needle and moxa *Zhou Lao* (LI 12), and *Chi Zi* (Lu 5).

(23) **Both shoulder blades painful:** Needle and moxa *Jian Jing* (GB 21), and *Zhi Gou* (TH 6).

(24) **Wrist pain:** Moxa *Yang Xi* (LI 5), *Qu Chi* (LI 11), and *Wan Gu* (SI 4).

(25) **Elbow, forearm, and wrist pain:** Needle *Qian Gu* (SI 2), *Ye Men* (TH 2), and *Zhong Zhu* (TH 3).

18) *ZU* (Foot/Lower Limb)

(1) **Leg/knee spasm (and) pain:** Needle and/or moxa *Feng Shi* (GB 31), *Yang Ling Quan* (GB 34), *Qu Quan* (Liv 8), and *Kun Lun* (Bl 60).

(2) **Thigh/shin acute pain:** Needle and/or moxa *Feng Shi* (GB 31), *Zhong Du* (GB 32), *Yang Jiao* (GB 35), *Xuan Zhong* (GB 39).

(3) **Leg flaccid, cannot contract:** Needle or moxa *Fu Liu* (Ki 7).

(4) **Knee painful, leg collapses**: Needle and/or moxa *Huan Tiao* (GB 30), *Xuan Zhong* (GB 39), *Ju Liao* (GB 29), and *Wei Zhong* (Bl 40).

(5) **Thigh pain, shin ache:** Needle and/or moxa *Yang Ling Quan* (GB 34), *Jue Gu* (GB 39), *Zhong Feng* (Liv 4), *Zu Lin Qi* (GB 41), *Zu San Li* (St 36), and *Yang Fu* (GB 38).

(6) **Pain (on the) inside of the knee:** Needle *Xi Guan* (Liv 7), *Tai Chong* (Liv 3), and *Zhong Feng* (Liv 4).

(7) **Pain (on the) outside of the knee:** Needle *Xia Xi* (GB 43), *Yang Jiao* (GB 35), and *Yang Ling* (GB 34).

(8) **Ankle pain:** Needle and/or moxa *Kun Lun* (Bl 60), *Tai Xi* (Ki 3), *Shen Mai* (Bl 62), *Qiu Xu* (GB 40), *Shang Qiu* (Sp 5), *Zhao Hai* (Ki 6), *Tai Chong* (Liv 3), and *Jie Xi* (St 41).

(9) **Extreme pain of the toes:** Needle and/or moxa *Yong Quan* (Ki 1) and *Ran Gu* (Ki 2).

(10) **Inside of knee painful:** Needle *Du Bi* (St 35).

Comment: We understand this to mean inside under the patella and not to mean the medial side.

(11) **Knee swollen:** Use fire needle puncture at *Zu San Li* (St 36), and then puncture *Xing Jian* (Liv 2).

(12) **Foot weak, emaciated, and cracked:** Needle and/or moxa *San Li* (St 36) and *Jue Gu* (GB 39).

(13) **Both legs (feel) like ice:** Moxa *Yin Shi* (St 33).

(14) **Pain (from the) lumbus (to the) sole:** Needle and/or

37

moxa *Huan Tiao* (GB 30), *Feng Shi* (GB 31), *Yin Shi* (St 33), *Wei Zhong* (Bl 40), *Cheng Shan* (Bl 57), *Kun Lun* (Bl 60), and *Shen Mai* (Bl 62).

(15) **Pain (on the) inside (of the) thigh (and) knee:** Needle *Wei Zhong* (Bl 40), *San Li* (St 36), and *San Yin Jiao* (Sp 6).

(16) **Leg (and) knees sore (and) painful:** Needle *Huan Tiao* (GB 30), *San Li* (St 36), *Yang Ling* (GB 34), and *Qiu Xu* (GB 40).

(17) **Foot (and) knee pain:** Needle *Wei Zhong* (Bl 40), *San Li* (St 36), *Qu Quan* (Liv 8), *Yang Ling* (GB 34), *Feng Shi* (GB 31), *Kun Lun* (Bl 60), and *Jie Xi* (St 41).

(18) **Foot (and) shin senseless (like a piece of) wood:** Needle *Haun Tiao* (GB 30) and *Feng Shi* (GB 31).

(19) **Paralysis of the leg:** Needle and/or moxa *Huan Tiao* (GB 30), *Yin Ling* (Sp 9), *Yang Fu* (GB 38), *Tai Xi* (Ki 3), and *Zhi Yin* (Bl 67).

(20) **Thigh pivot pain:** Choose *Huan Tiao* (GB 30), *Yang Ling* (GB 34), and *Qiu Xu* (GB 40).

Comment: Thigh pivot refers to the lateral aspect of the thigh around the prominence of the femur, i.e., the acetabulum.

(21) **Feet cold (and) hot:** Needle *San Li* (St 36), *Wei Zhong* (Bl 40), *Yang Ling* (GB 34), *Fu Liu* (Ki 7), *Ran Gu* (Ki 2), *Xing Jian* (Liv 2), *Zhong Feng* (Liv 4), *Da Du* (Sp 2), and *Yin Bai* (Sp 1).

(22) **Feet cold like ice:** Moxa *Shen Shu* (Bl 23).

(23) **Shin sore:** Moxa *Cheng Shan* (Bl 57) and *Jin Men* (Bl 63).

(24) **Foot (and) shin cold:** Needle and/or moxa *Fu Liu* (Ki 7), *Shen Mai* (Bl 62), and *Li Dui* (St 45).

(25) **Spasm of the leg:** Needle and/or moxa *Shen Shu* (Bl 23), *Yin Ling* (Sp 9), *Yang Fu* (GB 38), and *Jue Gu* (GB 39).

(26) **Swollen feet:** Needle and/or moxa *Cheng Shan* (Bl 57), *Kun Lun* (Bl 60), *Ran Gu* (Ki 2), *Wei Zhong* (Bl 40), *Xia Lian* (LI 8), and *Feng Shi* (GB 31).

(27) **Swollen legs:** Needle and/or moxa *Cheng Shan* (Bl 57) and *Kun Lun* (Bl 60).

(28) **Leg slack:** Needle and/or moxa *Yang Ling* (GB 34), *Jue Gu* (GB 39), *Tai Chong* (Liv 3), and *Qiu Xu* (GB 40).

(29) **Feet feeble or weak:** Needle and/or moxa *Wei Zhong* (Bl 40), *San Li* (St 36), and *Cheng Shan* (Bl 57).

(30) **Both knees red, swollen, (and) painful:** Needle and/or moxa *Xi Guan* (Liv 7), *Wei Zhong* (Bl 40), *Yang Fu* (GB 38), *San Yin Jiao* (Sp 6), *Fu Liu* (Ki 7), *Chong Yang* (St 42), *Ran Gu* (Ki 2), *Shen Mai* (Bl 62), *Xing Jian* (Liv 2), and *Pi Shu* (Bl 20).

(31) **Foot (and) ankle sore:** Needle and/or moxa *Wei Zhong* (Bl 40) and *Kun Lun* (Bl 60).

(32) **Pain (in the) center of the foot:** Needle and/or moxa *Kun Lun* (Bl 60).

(33) **Foot sinew twisted:** Needle or moxa *Cheng Shan* (Bl 57).

(34) **Foot qi:** Moxa in sequence *Feng Fu* (GV 16), *Fu Tiu* (St 32), *Du Bi* (St 35), *San Li* (St 36), *Shang Lian* (LI 9), *Xia Lian* (LI 8), and *Jue Gu* (GB 39). Moxa these in sequence.

19) *PI* (Skin)

(1) **Vitiligo:** Moxa 3-5 cones on the palmar side of the middle finger of both hands, inside the crease dividing the finger from the hand.

(2) **Scrofulous sores:** Same as above.

(3) **(Feeling) like worms are crawling all over the body:** Moxa elbow tip 7 cones; needle *Qu Chi* (LI 11), *Shen Men* (Ht 7), *He Gu* (LI 4), and *Zu San Li* (St 36).

20) *ROU* (Flesh)

(1) **Warts:** Moxa 3-5 cones on the palmar side of the middle finger of both hands, inside the crease dividing the finger from the hands. Then moxa 3-5 cones on *Zhi Zheng* (SI 7), and just above *Zhi Zheng* 3 to 5 cones.

21) *MAI* (Vessels)

Comment: The word *mai* may mean either vessels or pulse. In this context as one of a list of body parts, it must be listed as vessel.

(1) **Injury due to cold; six pulses gone:** Moxa seven cones each on *Fu Liu* (Ki 7), *He Gu* (LI 4), *Zhong Ji* (CV 3), *Zhi*

Gou (TH 6), *Ju Que* (CV 14), and *Qi Chong* (St 30). Also moxa profusely on *Qi Hai* (CV 6).

(2) **Ceaseless dry heaves, four limbs inversion chill, pulse severed:** Moxa 30 cones on *Jian Shi* (Per 5).

(3) **Condition of no pulse:** Needle and moxa on *Nei Guan* (Per 6), and *Tai Yuan* (Lu 9).

22) *JIN* (Sinews)

(1) **Sinews contracted and bones painful:** Needle and moxa *Hun Men* (Bl 47).

(2) **Knee bent; sinews taut and won't relax:** Needle and moxa *Qu Quan* (Liv 8).

(3) **Sinews taut, won't relax:** If the inner ankle bone sinew is stiff, moxa it 30 cones; if the outer ankle bone sinew is stiff, moxa it 30 cones.

(4) **Knee sinews urgently contracted and won't open:** Moxa 14 cones on *Wei Yang* (Bl 39).

(5) **Sinew pattern due to liver heat:** Tonify *Xing Jian* (Liv 2), disperse *Tai Chong* (Liv 3).

(6) **Sinews contracted, yin withdrawn:** Moxa 50 cones on *Zhong Feng* (Liv 4).

Comment: Yin here refers to the testicles.

(7) **Sinews twisted and painful:** Disperse *Cheng Shan* (Bl 57)

or moxa 14 cones.

(8) **Sinew *hui* point *Yang Ling Quan* (GB 34):** For wind sinew disease one should choose this point.

23) *GU* (Bones)

(1) **Spine stiff and painful:** Needle *Ren Zhong* (GV 26).

(2) **Sinews contracted, bone pain:** Needle and moxa *Hun Men* Bl 47).

(3) **Bones soft with no power:** Moxa *Da Shu* (Bl 11); (This is the *hui* point of the bones. This point is applicable for all bone diseases).

24) *QIAN YIN* (Front Yin, i.e., Genitalia)

(1) **Cold *shan* abdominal pain:** Moxa *Yin Shi* (St 33), *Tai Xi* (Ki 3), and *Gan Shu* (Bl 18).

Comment: Although often translated as hernia, Wiseman does not translate this term at all, preferring to leave it in Chinese. While the western term hernia is a type of *shan*, not all *shan* are hernias. We have therefore chosen to leave the term in Chinese *pin yin* except in those cases where it is clear from the text that a western diagnosis of hernia is what is actually being discussed.

(2) **Main method for all *shan*:** Choose *Da Dun* (Liv 1), *Xing Jian* (Liv 2), *Tai Chong* (Liv 3), *Zhong Feng* (Liv 4), *Li Gou* (Liv 5), *Guan Men* (St 22), *Guan Yuan* (CV 4), *Shui Dao* (St

29), *San Yin Jiao* (Sp 6), *Zu San Li* (St 36).

(3) *Shan* **causing testicular swelling and acute pain:** Choose *Li Gou* (Liv 5), *Da Dun* (Liv 1), *Yin Shi* (St 33), *Zao Hai* (Ki 6), *Xia Ju Xu* (St 39), *Xiao Chang Shu* (Bl 27).

(4) **Foxy** *shan*: Choose *Tai Chong* (Liv 3), *Gong Sun* (Sp 5), *Da Dun* (Liv 1), *Li Gou* (Liv 5).

Comment: Foxy or fox *shan* is when a part of the small intestine intermittently descends into the scrotum, but disappears when the person lies down.

(5) **Women's** *shan* **intermittent lump pain (Same as foxy** *shan* **in men):** Choose the same points as in number four above plus, needle *Tian Jing* (TH 10), also moxa *Qi Hai* (CV 6) and *Zhong Ji* (CV 3).

(6) **Ulcerous** *shan* **with prolapse to one side:** Choose *Da Ju* (St 27), *Di Ji* (Sp 3), *Zhong Ji* (CV 3), *Zhong Feng* (Liv 4), *Jiao Xin* (Ki 8), *Yong Quan* (Ki 1).

(7) **Water ulcer; single sided prolapse:** Choose *Lan Men* (appendix gate; 3 cun leteral to *Qu Gu* (CV 2), *San Yin Jiao* (Sp 6).

Comment: *Shui kui chuang* means a water ulcer. The word *chuang* was left out here.

(8) **Pediatric fetal** *shan*; **one-sided testicle:** Moxa 3 cones above the crease behind and above the scrotum. In spring (if you do) moxa, in summer (it will be) healed. (If you) moxa in summer, (the patient will) recover in winter.

Comment: This describes an undescended testicle in children

43

from birth.

(9) *Shan* **lump pain:** Moxa 3-5 cones on *Zhao Hai* (Ki 6). Needle and/or moxa *Yin Ling Quan* (Sp 9) and *Qiu Xu* (GB 40).

(10) **Sudden** *shan*: Needle and/or moxa *Qiu Xu* (GB 40), *Da Dun* (Liv 1), *Yin Shi* (St 33), *Xue Hai* (Sp 10).

(11) **One sided water** *shan*: Moxa *Gui Lai* (St 29), *Da Dun* (Liv 1), and *San Yin Jiao* (Sp 6).

Comment: This describes a hydrocele, where the skin is stretched and looks transparent.

(12) **Yin** *shan*: Moxa *Tai Chong* (Liv 3) and *Da Dun* (Liv 1).

Comment: Testicular *shan*.

(13) **Yin enter abdomen:** Moxa *Guan Yuan* (CV 4) and *Da Dun* (Liv 1).

Cooment: Undescended or retracted testicles.

(14) **Frequent urination:** Moxa *Shen Shu* (Bl 23) and *Guan Yuan* (CV 4).

(15) **Yin swelling:** Needle or moxa *Qu Quan* (Liv 8), *Tai Xi* (Ki 3), *Da Dun* (Liv 1), *Shen Shu* (Bl 23), *San Yin Jiao* (Sp 6).

Comment: Testicular swelling.

(16) **Penis pain:** Needle and/or moxa *Yin Ling Quan* (Sp 9), *Qu Quan* (Liv 8), *Xing Jian* (Liv 2), *Tai Chong* (Liv 3), *Yin Gu* (Ki 10), *Shen Shu* (Bl 23), *Zhong Ji* (CV 3), *San Yin Jiao*

(Sp 6), *Da Dun* (Liv 1), *Tai Xi* (Ki 3), etc.

(17) **Spermatorrhea:** Moxa *Shen Shu* (Bl 23).

(18) **Retroversion of the uterus, no drowning, *lin* dribbling:** Needle and moxa *Guan Yuan* (CV 4).

Comment: Drowning here implies a lack of copious free flow of the urine. *Lin* is a disease category which describes dribbling conditions.

(19) **White turbidity:** Needle and/or moxa *Shen Shu* (Bl 23), *Guan Yuan* (CV 4), and *San Yin Jiao* (Sp 6).

Comment: *Bai Zhuo* is a disease category in which there is turbid urine like swill or slops. This has to do with stomach turbid qi oozing down into the bladder being expelled by the bladder.

(20) **Cold and hot qi *lin*:** Needle *Yin Ling Quan* (Sp 9).

Comment: Qi *lin* is one of the *wu lin* or five *lin* which is *lin* due to stagnation of liver qi in the lower burner. The hot and cold here refers to the *shao yang* phase of disease which also relates to the liver. .

(21) **Urination yellow and red:** Needle *San Yin Jiao* (Sp 6), *Tai Xi* (Ki 3), *Shen Shu* (Bl 23), *Qi Hai* (CV 6), *Pang Guang Shu* (Bl 28), and *Guan Yuan* (CV 4).

Comment: Red urine means dark, not bloody.

(22) **Red urine with blood:** Needle *Da Ling* (Per 7), and *Guan Yuan* (CV 4).

(23) **Pain of the scrotum:** Needle *Zhong Feng* (Liv 4).

(24) **Bladder qi:** Needle and moxa *Wei Zhong* (Bl 40) and *Wei Yang* (Bl 39).

Comment: This means distention of the bladder.

(25) **Small intestine qi:** Moxa the following 7 cones each: *Feng Shi* (GB 31), *Qi Hai* (CV 6), *Tao Chong* (Liv 3), *Du Yin* (see note above section 15 #8). Also moxa *Wai Ling* on both sides of the navel, 1.5 cun to either side, each side 7 cones. This has an immediate effect.

Comment: The full description of this is *xiao chang qi shan* which specifically means hernia.

(26) **Miscellaneous *shan* with upward flushing of qi:** A miraculous effect is achieved by using moxa on *Du Yin*.

Comment: For the location of *Du Yin* see #8 under Section 15 on page 33.

(27) **Wooden kidney: enlarged rigid testicle with no pain:** Needle and moxa *Da Dun* (Liv 1), and *San Yin Jiao* (Sp 6).

Comment: Kidney here is the *wai shen* or external kidney which means the testicle.

(28) **Wooden kidney red and painful:** Needle *Ran Gu* (Kid 2) and *Lan Men* (extra point 3 cun lateral to CV 2).

(29) **Several kinds (miscellaneous) of *shan*:** Moxa 7 cones on *Guan Yuan* (CV 4) and 7 cones on *Da Dun* (Liv 1).

(30) *Shan* **moxa method:** Use a piece of straw to measure the

patient's mouth from corner to corner; use that measure piece to make a triangle. Place the top of the triangle on the center of the patient's umbilicus. The points will be at the tips of the other two corners on either side below the umbilicus. If the hernia is on one side, use moxa on the other side. This is called the triangle moxa method.

25) *HOU YIN* (Anus)

(1) **Hemorrhoid aching:** Needle/moxa *Cheng Shan* (Bl 57) and *Chang Qiang* (GV 1).

(2) **Hemorrhoid pain:** Needle/moxa *Cheng Jin* (Bl 56), *Fei Yang* (Bl 58), *Wei Zhong* (Bl 40), *Cheng Fu* (Bl 36), *Zhan Zhu* (Bl 2), *Hui Yin* (CV 1), *Shang Qiu* (Sp 5), etc.

(3) **Anal prolapse:** Needle/moxa *Da Chang Shu* (Bl 25), *Bai Hui* (GV 20), *Chang Qiang* (GV 1), *Jian Jing* (GB 21), *He Gu* (LI 4), and *Qi Chong* (St 30).

(4) **Hemorrhoid trickle:** Make a dough out of powdered *Fu Zi* (Radix Praeparatus Aconiti Carmichaeli) and saliva. Form small cakes and put one on the anus, lighting moxa on top of the cake to warm the area slightly. If the cake dries out, change to a fresh cake. Do this several times per day untilthe area becomes flat and smooth.

Comment: The word used here is *lou*, the same word as in *beng lou*. The implication is a leaking or intermittent bleeding.

(5) **Explosive/violent diarrhea:** Needle and moxa *Yin Bai* (Sp 1).

(6) **Dysentery/diarrhea:** Needle *Qu Quan* (Liv 8), *Tai Xi* (Ki 3), *Tai Bai* (Sp 3), *Pi Shu* (Bl 20), *Xiao Chang Shu* (Bl 27), and *Tai Chong* (Liv 3).

(7) **Blood in the feces:** Needle and moxa *Cheng Shan* (Bl 57), *Fu Liu* (Ki 7), *Tai Chong* (Liv 3) and *Tai Bai* (Sp 3).

(8) **Feces not controlled (incontinent):** Moxa *Da Chang Shu* (Bl 25) and *Guan Yuan* (CV 4).

(9) **Bleeding after defecation:** Needle and moxa *Cheng Shan* (Bl 57), *Jie Xi* (St 41), *Tai Bai* (Sp 3), and *Dai Mai* (GB 26).

(10) **Intestinal wind:** Moxa 100 cones at the place where the tail bone ends. [*Chang Qiang* (GV 1)].

Comment: Intestinal wind means bright bleeding during and preceeding the passage of stool.

(11) **Anal prolapse; (anus) not contracted:** Moxa seven cones at *Bai Hui* (GV 20) and *Wei Jiu* (tip of the tailbone); moxa on the navel as many cones as the person is years old.

(12) **Bleeding hemorrhoids:** Moxa *Cheng Shan* (Bl 57) and *Fu Liu* (Ki 7).

(13) **Longterm hemorrhoids:** Moxa *Er Bai* (an extra point for hemorrhoids located 4 cun above the carpal crease on both sides of the tendon flexor carpi radialis, i.e. two points on each arm), *Cheng Shan* (Bl 57), and *Chang Qiang* (GV 1).

Hemorrhoid moxa method, apart from the above treatments: Moxa on the center of the navel and one inch apart from the center of the navel on each side. Moxa seven cones on each.

3

Miscellaneous Conditions

1) *FENG* (Wind)

(1) **Wind stroke with abundant phlegm, voice is raspy:** *Qi Hai* (CV 6), *Guan Yuan* (CV 4). Moxa each one 200-300 cones. There will probably be a response (to this treatment).

(2) **Sudden wind stroke with deviation of the mouth and drooling:** Moxa *Ting Hui* (GB 2), *Jia Che* (St 6), *Di Cang* (St 4), *Bai Hui* (GV 20), *Jian Yu* (Li 15), *Qu Chi* (LI 11), *Feng Shi* (GB 31), *Zu San Li* (St 36), *Xuan Zhong* (GB 39), the lower border of the hairline in front of the ear, *Da Zhui* (GV 14), *Feng Chi* (GB 20), etc.

(3) **Wind stroke with the eyes staring up (rolling back in the head):** Moxa *Si Zhu Kong* (TH 23), the second vertebra and the fifth vertebra, 7 cones each. Set them on fire simultaneously.

(4) **Mouth and eyes both deviated:** Moxa *Ting Hui* (GB 2), *Jia Che* (St 6), *Di Cang* (St 4). Find the depression in the middle of the cheeks; if the mouth is pulled to one side, moxa the cheek in that depression on the other side, and vice versa.

(5) **One-sided paralysis (hemiplegia):** Moxa *Bai Hui* (GV 20),

Xin Hui (GV 22), *Feng Chi* (GB 20), *Jian Yu* (LI 15), *Qu Chi* (LI 11), *He Gu* (LI 4), *Huan Tiao* (GB 30), *Zu San Li* (St 36), *Feng Shi* (GB 31) and *Jue Gu* (GB 39).

(6) **Mouth silent; cannot speak (lockjaw):** Needle *Ren Zhong* (GV 26), *He Gu* (LI 4), *Jia Che* (St 6), and *Bai Hui* (GV 20); or moxa *Yi Feng* (TH 17).

(7) **Unable to speak:** Needle *Ya Men* (GV 15), *Ren Zhong* (GV 26), *Tian Tu* (CV 22), *Yong Quan* (Ki 1), *Shen Men* (Ht 7), *Zhi Gou* (TH 6), *Feng Fu* (GV 16), etc.

(8) **Back turned as it is would break (opisthotonis):** Needle *Ya Men* (GV 15) and *Feng Fu* (GV 16).

(9) **Wind epilepsy/sudden epilepsy:** Needle/moxa *Feng Chi* (GB 20), *Bai Hui* (GV 20), *Chih Ze* (Lu 5), and *Shao Chong* (Ht 9).

(10) **Omens of wind stroke of the *fu* bowels:** Four limbs tingling and sore continuing for a long time before it diminishes. This is an indication of wind stroke to the bowels. In case of this symptom moxa *Bai Hui* (GV 20), *Qu Chi* (LI 11), *Feng Shi* (GB 31), *San Li* (St 36) and *Jue Gu* (GB 39).

11) **Omens of wind stroke in the *zang* organs:** The person will always feel anxious, the spirit is not regulated or calm, and the four limbs are numb. In this case moxa *Bai Hui* (GV 20), *Feng Chi* (GB 20), *Da Zhui* (GV 14), *Jian Jing* (GB 21), *Qu Chi* (LI 11), *Jian Shi* (Per 5), and *San Li* (St 36).

(12) **Bone *bi*:** Needle and/or moxa *Tai Xi* (Ki 3) and *Wai Zhong* (Bl 40).

Comment: While *bi* is another term which is often left

untranslated, in #12 through #16 it relates to the wind obstructing or blocking the normal flow of qi and blood in various levels of tissues in the body.

(13) **Sinew** *bi*: Needle and/or moxa *Tai Chong* (Liv 3) and *Yang Ling Quan* (GB 34).

(14) **Vessel** *bi*: Needle and/or moxa *Da Ling* (Per 7) and *Shao Hai* (Ht 3).

(15) **Flesh** *bi*: Needle and/or moxa *Tai Bai* (Sp 3) and *San Li* (St 36).

(16) **Skin** *bi*: Needle and/or moxa *Tai Yuan* (Lu 9) and *He Gu* (LI 4). In *bi* diseases it is suitable to use a hot needle to prick swiftly and repeatedly until the patient can feel it. Use the most tender spot as the point. It is believed that acupuncture should continue until the patient responds. The tender spot is always the point to use, it is not necessary to use regular meridian points.

(17) **Rheumatism/rheumatic arthritis:** Use the above described method, also moxa 21 cones on the *a-shi* point(s) and that will be excellent.

(18) **The 100 joints sore and disabled with no sensation:** Pierce *Jue Gu* (GB 39) with a triangular needle to release some blood.

2) *HAN* (Cold)

(1) **Cold injury:** On the first and second day (if there is) headache and high fever, it is appropriate to moxa *Ju Que*

(CV 14), *Shang Wan* (CV 13), *Zhong Wan* (CV 12) 50 cones on each (point).

(2) **Cold injury with headache; hot and cold:** (On the) first day needle *Feng Fu* (GV 16); (on the) second day needle *Nei Ting* (St 44); (on the) third day needle *Zu Lin Qi* (GB 41); (on the) fourth day needle *Yin Bai* (Sp 1); (on the) fifth day needle *Tai Xi* (Ki 3); (on the) sixth day needle *Zhong Feng* (Liv 4). (If the disease remains) on the outside, pierce the three yang channel points. (If the disease remains) on the inside, pierce the three yin channel points. (If) six days have passed (and the pathogen) has passed through (all the) channels (but still there is) no sweat, needle *Qi Men* (Liv 14).

The above mentioned first day, second day, etc. do not necessarily refer to the exact number of days. If the pathogen lingers in the *tai yang*, (then it is usual to) pierce *Feng Fu* (GV 16); in the *yang ming* (then it is usual to) pierce *Nei Ting* (St 44); in the *shao yang* (then) pierce *Zu Lin Qi* (GB 41). If a week passes and the pathogen goes through all the channels (levels) without (the patient) sweating, puncture *Qi Men* (Liv 14). In the treatment of cold injury, nothing other than the 3 big methods of sweating, vomiting, and purging (are used). Today we will deal with these as follows:

(3) **Cold injury with unremittent high fever:** Needle *Qu Chi* (LI 11), *Jue Gu* (GB 39), *Xian Gu* (St 43): supplementary points (could be) *Er Jian* (LI 2), *Nei Ting* (St 44), *Qian Gu* (SI 2), *Tong Gu* (Bl 66), *Ye Men* (TH 2), and *Xia Xi* (GB 43).

(4) **Cold injury headache:** Needle *Zan Zhu* (Bl 2) and *He Gu* (LI 4).

(5) **Cold injury (with) no sweating:** Needle *He Gu* (LI 4), *Fu Liu* (Ki 7), *Wang Gu* (SI 4), *Yang Gu* (SI 5), *Xia Xi* (GB 43),

Li Dui (St 45), *Lao Gong* (Per 8), *Feng Chi* (GB 20), *Yu Ji* (Lu 10), *Jing Qu* (Lu 8), *Nei Ting* (St 44), and *Er Jian* (LI 2); for supplementary points pierce the *jing* well points of all 12 channels.

Comment: To create sweating, see #2 on page 8.

(6) **Cold injury (with) excessive sweating:** Needle *He Gu* (LI 4), *Fu Liu* (Ki 7), and *Nei Ting* (St 44).

Comment: To stop sweating, see #1 on page 8.

(7) *Tai yang* **pattern headache due to cold injury:** Needle *Tou Wan Gu* (GB 12), and *Jing Gu* (Bl 64).

(8) *Yang ming* **pattern headache due to cold injury:** Needle *He Gu* (LI 4), and *Chong Yang* (St 42).

(9) *Shao yang* **pattern headache due to cold injury:** Needle *Yang Chi* (TH 4), *Qiu Xu* (GB 40), *Feng Fu* (GV 16), and *Feng Chi* (GB 20).

(10) **Cold injury chest bind:** First knead (rub) the left side of the painful area below the zyphoid process; then punture the left side with filiform needles; follow this by puncturing *Zhi Gou* (TH 6) and *Jian Shi* (Per 5) on the right side. On the right side repeat the whole procedure as described above. (While having the patient) breathe slowly and gently, stop needling. The effect is instant.

(11) **Cold injury yin condition abdominal pain:** Moxa on the outer side of the small toe, on the lateral end of the most proximal crease. On a man (use the) left side; on a woman, the right side.

(12) **Cold injury chest pain:** Needle *Qi Men* (Liv 14) and *Da Ling* (Per 7).

(13) **Cold injury flank pain:** Needle *Zhi Gou* (TH 6) and *Yang Ling Quan* (GB 34).

(14) **Cold injury body hot:** Needle *Xian Gu* (St 43), *Lu Xi* (nickname for *Tai Xi*) (Ki 3), *Shou San Li* (LI 10), *Fu Liu* (Ki 7), *Xia Xi* (GB 43), *Gong Sun* (Sp 4), *Tai Bai* (Sp 3), *Wei Zhong* (Bl 40), and *Yong Quan* (Ki 1).

(15) **Cold injury hot and cold:** Needle *Feng Chi* (GB 20), *Shao Hai* (Ht 3), *Yu Ji* (Lu 10), *Shao Chong* (Ht 9), *He Gu* (LI 4), *Fu Liu* (Ki 7), *Zu Lin Qi* (GB 41), and *Tai Bai* (Sp 3).

(16) **Cold injury lingering residual fever:** Needle *Qu Chi* (LI 11), *Zu San Li* (St 36), *He Gu* (LI 4), *Nei Ting* (St 44), and *Tai Chong* (Liv 3).

(17) **Cold injury constipation:** Needle *Zhao Hai* (Ki 6) and *Zhang Men* (Liv 13).

(18) **Cold injury urine not free flowing:** Needle *Yin Gu* (Ki 10) and *Yin Ling Quan* (Sp 9).

(19) **Cold injury mania:** Needle *Bai Lao* (M-HN-30) extra point), *Jian Shi* (Per 5), *He Gu* (LI 4) and *Fu Liu* (Ki 7).

(20) **Cold injury; unaware of human affairs (loss of consciousness):** Needle *Zhong Zhu* (TH 3) and *Zu San Li* (St 36).

(21) **Yin toxins (potentially dangerous) due to cold injury:** Moxa 200 to 300 cones on the navel; also moxa 200 to 300 cones on *Qi Hai* (CV 6) and *Guan Yuan* (CV 4).

(22) **Yin pattern shrunken (contracted) penis due to cold injury:** With the help of an assistant to hold it erect, moxa 3 cones at the opening.

(23) **Cold injury; disappearance of the 6 pulses:** Moxa *Fu Liu* (Ki 7), *He Gu* (LI 4), *Zhong Ji* (CV 3), *Zhi Gou* (TH 6), *Ju Que* (CV 14), and *Qi Chong* (St 30).

(24) **Hands and feet inversion chill:** Moxa *Da Du* (Sp 2).

(25) **Recurrent heat after the subsiding of a fever in a cold injury:** Needle *Feng Men* (Bl 12), *He Gu* (LI 4), *Xing Jian* (Liv 2), and *Jue Gu* (GB 39).

(26) **Sorrow, fear due to cold injury:** Needle *Tai Chong* (Liv 3), *Nei Ting* (St 44), *Shao Chong* (Ht 9), and *Tong Li* (Ht 5).

(27) **Cold injury stiffness at the neck; eyes closed:** Needle *Feng Men* (Bl 12), *Wei Zhong* (Bl 40), *Tai Chong* (Liv 3), *Nei Ting* (St 44), *Zu San Li* (St 36), and *San Yin Jiao* (Sp 6).

(28) **Opisthotonis:** First needle *Tian Tu* (CV 22); next needle *Shan Zhong* (CV 17), *Tai Chong* (Liv 3), *Gan Shu* (Bl 18), *Wei Zhong* (Bl 40), *Kun Lun* (Bl 60), *Da Zhui* (Bl 14), and *Bai Hui* (GV 20).

(29) **Puncturing method of the 59 vertebrae in cases of hot disease due to cold injury:** Application of the five points located on the five lines on the scalp (from medial to lateral) is used to control rebellious heat of the several yang meridians. The central line on the head (consists of) *Shang Xing* (GV 23), *Xin Hui* (GV 22), *Qian Ding* (GV 21), *Bai Hui* (GV 20), and *Hou Ding* (GV 19). (These are) flanked by *tai yang jing Cheng Guang* (Bl 6), *Tong Tian* (Bl 7), *Luo Que* (Bl

8), *Yu Zhen* (Bl 9), and *Tian Zhu* (Bl 10). Again flanked by *shao yang jing Tou Lin Qi* (GB 15), *Mu Chuang* (GB 16), *Zheng Ying* (GB 17), *Cheng Ling* (GB 18), and *Nao Kong* (GB 19). To purge heat in the middle use *Da Zhu* (Bl 11), *Du Shu* (Bl 16), *Que Pen* (St 12), and *Bei Shu* (another name for *Feng Men* [Bl 12]), *Qi Chong* (St 30), *Zu San Li* (St 36), *Shang Ju Xu* (St 37), and *Xia Ju Xu* (St 39) respectively are used to clear heat from the stomach.

3) *SHI* (Damp)

In Damp diseases use moxa. This will promote the free flow of the meridians and circulation of qi in the meridians. Only in *bi* syndromes and damp heat cases, athletes foot, and flaccidity (*wei)* syndromes it is preferrable to use needles.

4) *HUO* (Fire)

(1) **Steaming bone consumptive heat:** Moxa *San Li* (St 36) and *Gao Huang Shu* (Bl 43); if the person is still not emaciated or deformed moxa *Hua Xue* (Bl 17 and Bl 19).

(2) **Body hot, taxing cough:** Moxa *Po Hu* (Bl 42).

(3) **Both hands great heat as if on fire:** Moxa 3-5 cones on *Yong Quan* (Ki 1).

(4) **Dry front teeth due to steaming bone disease:** Moxa *Da Zhui* (GV 14).

(5) **Body hot like fire, feet chilly like ice:** Moxa *Yang Fu* (GB 38).

(6) **Heart vexation:** Needle *Shen Men* (Ht 7), *Yang Xi* (LI 5), *Wan Gu* (SI 4), *Shao Shang* (Lu 11), *Jie Xi* (St 41), *Gong Sun* (Sp 4), *Tai Bai* (Sp 3), and *Zhi Yin* (Bl 67).

(7) **Vexation and thirst; heat in the heart:** Needle *Qu Ze* (Per 3).

(8) **Heart vexation and racing:** Needle *Yu Ji* (Lu 10).

(9) **Empty vexation, dry mouth:** Needle or moxa *Fei Shu* (Bl 13).

(10) **Vexation, oppression, cannot lie down:** Needle or moxa *Tai Yuan* (Lu 9), *Gong Sun* (Sp 4), *Yin Bai* (Sp 1), *Fei Shu* (Bl 13), *Yin Ling Quan* (Sp 9), and *San Yin Jiao* (Sp 6).

Comment: The Chinese word *men* is translated here as oppression. *Men* suggests the image of something tightly covered up, smothered, and shut in. It also can be translated as stuffy.

(11) **Stomach heat; cannot eat:** Needle or moxa *Xia Lian* (LI 8).

(12) **Somnolence with reluctance to speak:** Needle or moxa *Ge Shu* (Bl 17).

(13) **Stomach heat:** Needle or moxa *Jue Gu* (GB 39).

5) *NEI SHANG* (Internal Injury)

(1) **Stomach weakness; indifference to food and drink:** Needle and moxa *Zu San Li* (St 36) and *San Yin Jiao* (Sp 6).

(2) **Evil heat in the triple heater; no desire to eat:** Moxa *Guan Yuan* (CV 4).

(3) **No thought of food or drink:** Bleed *Ran Gu* (Ki 2).

(4) **Hunger but unable to eat; food and drink won't go down the throat:** Needle and moxa *Zhang Men* (Liv 13) and *Qi Men* (Liv 14).

(5) **Appetite reduced, heart and abdomen inflated and distented; face withered and yellowish:** [This is a type of ascariasis spread by mosquitoes where rice is grown. It attacks the liver. It still occurs in the countryside in China. A person suffering this has a waxy complexion, and is emaciated except for the extremely bloated belly.] Needle and moxa *Zhong Wan* (CV 12).

(6) **Eating much; body remains skinny:** First select *Pi Shu* (Bl 20) and later use *Zhang Men* (Liv 13) and *Tai Chang* (nickname for CV 12).

(7) **Food won't descend; diaphragm blockage; not free flowing:** Evil in the stomach and abdomen. Needle and moxa *Shang Wan* (CV 13) and *Xia Wan* (CV 10).

(8) **Stomach disease; food won't go down:** Needle and moxa *Zu San Li* (St 36).

(9) **Vomiting food eaten the night before, acid regurgitation, and noisy, upset stomach:** Use *Zhang Men* (Liv 13) and *Shen Lan* (extra point, no references available).

6) *XU LAO* (Empty Taxation)

(1) **The five consumptive diseases:** Needle and/or moxa *Zu San Li* (St 36).

(2) **Body hot, taxing cough:** Needle and/or moxa *Po Hu* (Bl 42).

(3) **Empty taxation steaming bone night sweat:** Needle and/or moxa *Yin Xi* (Ht 6).

(4) **Insufficient true qi:** Moxa *Qi Hai* (CV 6).

(5) **100 types (any kind) of empty taxation:** Moxa *Gao Huang Shu* (Bl 43), *Si Hua Xue* (Bl 17 & Bl 19), and *Yao Shu* (GV 2). This treatment is best for patients with emptiness of yang qi.

7) *KE CHUAN* (Cough and Wheezing, Dyspnea)

(1) **Cough with phlegm:** Needle or moxa *Tian Tu* (CV 22), *Fei Shu* (Bl 13), and *Feng Long* (St 40).

(2) **Cough with rising qi and much vomiting of chilly phlegm:** Moxa 50 cones on *Fei Shu* (Bl 13).

(3) **Cough, voice damaged, throat hoarse:** Needle and/or moxa *Tian Tu* (CV 22).

(4) **Longterm trouble with cough and wheezing, inability to sleep:** Moxa *Gao Huang Shu* (Bl 43).

(5) **Longterm cough:** Moxa *Fei Shu* (Bl 13) and *Gao Huang*

Shu (Bl 43).

(6) **Cold injury severe cough:** Moxa 14 cones on *Tian Tu* (CV 22).

(7) **Dyspnea tension:** Moxa *Fei Shu* (Bl 13), *Tian Tu* (CV 22), and *Zu San Li* (St 36).

(8) **Asthmatic wheezing:** Moxa all of the following points: *Fei Shu* (Bl 13), *Tian Tu* (CV 21), *Shan Zhong* (CV 17), *Fei Shu* (Bl 13), *Xuan Ji* (CV 22), *Shu Fu* (Ki 27), *Ru Gen* (St 18), and *Qi Hai* (CV 6).

(9) **Cough, wheezing; unable to lie down:** Needle *Yun Men* (Lu 2) and *Tai Yuan* (Lu 9).

(10) **Stuffy wheezing, phlegm fullness:** Needle *Tai Xi* (Ki 3) and *Feng Long* (St 40).

(11) **Qi counterflow with foul odor:** Needle *Shan Zhong* (CV 17), *Zhong Wan* (CV 12), *Fei Shu* (Bl 13), *Zu San Li* (St 36), and *Xing Jian* (Liv 2).

(12) **Qi counterflow:** Moxa *Zhong Wan* (CV 12), *Shan Zhong* (CV 17), *Qi Men* (Liv 14), and *Guan Yuan* (CV 4); also moxa *Zhi Gu Xue,* an extra point found 1 cun below the center of the nipple in the 5th intercostal space.

(13) **Incessant counterflow cough:** Moxa *Ru Gen* (St 18) 2 cones, or moxa *Qi Hai* (CV 6) or *Da Zhui* (GV 14) the same number of cones as years of age. If the patient can sleep only in a lateral recumbent posture and cannot lie or sleep on the back then moxa *San Yin Jiao* (Sp 6). Use the left side if the patient can lie only on the right side and vice versa.

(14) **Cough:** Needle and/or moxa *Lie Que* (Lu 7), *Jing Qu* (Lu 8), *Chi Ze* (Lu 5), *Zu San Li* (St 36), *Kun Lun* (Bl 60), *Fei Shu* (Bl 13), etc.

(15) **Cough with radiating pain in the flanks:** Needle or moxa *Gan Shu* (Bl 18).

(16) **Cough with pain in the lumbar vertebra:** Needle *Yu Ji* (Lu 10).

(17) **Technique to end asthma completely:** Using a piece of string, make a loop and put it over the neck. Tighten the loop to just fit around the middle of the neck and measure the end of the string to the tip of the ziphoid process. Then, keeping this measurement, pull the end of the string around to the back of the neck and where it touches on either side is the place to moxa.

Comment: This location sounds like an ancient method of finding *Ding Chuan* the extra point located .5 to 1 *cun* lateral to the spinous process of the 7th cervical vertebrae.

8) *OU TU* (Vomiting)

(1) **Tendency to vomit bitter water:** Needle *Zu San Li* (St 36) and *Yang Ling Quan* (GB 34).

(2) **Vomiting; food not digested/transformed:** Needle or moxa *Shang Wan* (CV 13), *Zhong Wan* (CV 12), and *Xia Wan* (CV 10).

(3) **Stomach reflux:** Moxa 100 cones on *Gao Huang Shu* (Bl 43); moxa 7 cones on *Shan Zhong* (CV 17) and *Zu San Li* (St

36); also moxa *Jian Jing* (GB 21) 5 to 7 cones.

(4) **Morning food vomited in the evening:** Moxa *Xin Shu* (Bl 15), *Ge Shu* (Bl 17), *Shan Zhong* (CV 17), *Ju Que* (CV 14), and *Zhong Wan* (CV 12).

(5) **Five chokes; five belches:** Needle and/or moxa *Tian Tu* (CV 22), *Shan Zhong* (CV 17), *Xin Shu* (Bl 15), *Shang Wan* (CV 13), *Zhong Wan* (CV 12), *Xia Wan* (CV 10), *Pi Shu* (Bl 20), *Wei Shu* (Bl 21), *Tong Guan* (no references available), *Zhong Wan* (CV 12), *Da Ling* (Per 7), and *Zu San Li* (St 36).

Comment: No references are available describing this concept, but analyzing the point indicates the treatment of counterflow and bound qi possibly due to food stagnation.

(6) **Vomiting unable to eat:** Needle and/or moxa from among *Qu Ze* (Per 3), *Tong Li* (Ht 5), *Lao Gong* (Per 8), *Yang Ling Quan* (GB 34), *Tai Xi* (Ki 3), *Zhao Hai* (Ki 6), *Tai Chong* (Liv 3), *Da Du* (Sp 2), *Yin Bai* (Sp 1), *Tong Gu* (Ki 20), *Wei Shu* (Bl 21), and *Fei Shu* (Bl 13).

(7) **Counterflow retching:** Needle or moxa *Da Ling* (Per 7).

(8) **Vomiting of fetid:** Needle *Tai Yuan* (Lu 9).

(9) **Dry heaves without intensity but ceaseless:** Moxa 3 cones on *Chi Ze* (Lu 5), and *Da Ling* (Per 7).

9) *ZHANG MAN* (Distension and Fullness)

(1) **Abdomen inside swollen and distended:** Needle or moxa *Nei Ting* (St 44).

(2) **Simple abdominal distention:** Needle *Shui Fen* (CV 9) 1 and 1/2 *cun*, moxa *Fu Liu* (Ki 7) 50 cones, moxa *San Yin Jiao* (Sp 6), and needle *Fu Liu* (Ki 7), *Zhong Feng* (Liv 4), and *Gong Sun* (Sp 4).

(3) **Distention and fullness:** Either needle or moxa *Zhong Wan* (CV 12), and *San Li* (St 36). In every case of distention always choose *San Li* (St 36), as distention demands (the use of this) point. Also choose *Zhong Wan* (CV 12) and *Qi Hai* (CV 6). Needle or moxa these points.

(4) **Heart abdomen distended and full:** Needle or moxa *Jue Gu* (GB 39) or *Nei Ting* (St 44).

(5) **Stomach and abdomen swollen and distended with loud gas:** Needle *He Gu* (LI 4), *San Li* (St 36), and *Qi Men* (Liv 14).

(6) **Water swelling:** Choose *Pian Li* (LI 6).

(7) **Swelling and distention:** Needle to a depth of 2 *cun* and 2 *fen* just above, below, to the right and to the left of the umbilicus.

(8) **Abdomen hard and large:** Needle and/or moxa *San Li* (St 36), *Yin Ling Quan* (Sp 9), *Qiu Xu* (GB 40), *Jie Xi* (St 41), *Qi Men* (Liv 14), *Chong Yang* (St 42), *Shui Fen* (CV 9), *Shen Que* (CV 8), and *Pang Guang Shu* (Bl 28).

(9) **Lower abdomen distended and full:** Needle *Zhong Feng* (Liv 4), *Ran Gu* (Ki 2) *Nei Ting* (St 44), and *Da Dun* (Liv 1).

10) *FU ZHONG* (Superficial Edema)

(1) **Turbidity (in the) body leads to edema, face puffy and enlarged:** Needle *Qu Chi* (LI 11), *He Gu* (LI 4), *San Li* (St 36), *Nei Ting* (St 44), *Xing Jian* (Liv 2), and *San Yin Jiao* (Sp 6). Moxa 3 cones on *Huai Xia* (Ankle Below), an extra point found below the medial malleolus at the edge of the red and white skin.

(2) **Superficial edema of the four limbs, face, and eyes:** Needle *Zhao Hai* (Ki 6), *Ren Zhong* (GV 26), *He Gu* (LI 4), *San Li* (St 36), *Jue Gu* (GB 39), *Qu Chi* (LI 11), *Zhong Wan* (CV 12), *Wan Gu* (SI 4), *Pi Shu* (Bl 20), *Wei Shu* (Bl 21), *Da Chang Shu* (Bl 25), *Pang Guang Shu* (Bl 28), and *San Yin Jiao* (Sp 6).

(3) **Superficial edema, swelling and distention:** Needle and/or moxa *Pi Shu* (Bl 20), *Wei Shu* (Bl 21), *Da Chang Shu* (Bl 25), *Pang Guang Shu* (Bl 28), *Shui Fen* (CV 9), *Zhong Wan* (CV 12), *San Li* (St 36), and *Xiao Chang Shu* (Bl 27).

(4) **Water swelling and qi distention and fullness:** Needle *Fu Liu* (Ki 7) and *Shen Que* (CV 8).

Comment: Although the text makes no mention of it, *Shen Que*, located at the navel, is classically forbidden to needle. Quite possibly it is an oversight and the text should read that this point is to be moxaed.

(5) **Four extremities, also the face, chest, abdomen, or any type of superficial edema or puffiness:** Moxa 100 cones on *Shui Fen* (CV 9) and *Qi Hai* (CV 6).

11) *JI JU* (Accumulations and Lumps)

(1) **Heart stagnation lump floating beam:** Needle and/or moxa *Shang Wan* (CV 13) and *San Li* (St 36).

Comment: Floating beam refers to a condition where there is a mass between the umbilicus and the zyphoid process which is hard and verticle like a roof beam. One of the *wu ji* or five lumps or stagnations.

(2) *Fei qi* **lung lump (aka)** *xi ben,* **inverted cup:** Needle or moxa *Ju Que* (CV 14) and *Qi Men* (Liv 14).

Comment: One of the *wu ji* or five abdominal lumps categorized by five phase correspondences. For a fuller discussion see "Wu Ji, The Five Accumulations", Flaws, Bob, *Australian Journal of Acupuncture, #* 14, Dec. '90, page 5-8.

(3) **Kidney accumulation running piggy:** Needle or moxa *Zhong Ji* (CV 3). Also moxa 100 cones on *Qi Hai* (CV 6), 3 cones on *Qi Men* (Liv 14), and 5 cones on *Du Yin* ([M-LE-18a] extra point, see page 33, #8 for location).

Comment: Running piggy is a translation for either the term *ben tun* or *shen ji*, one of the five accumulations, several of which are being described in this section. These terms describe a condition in which there is a lump or accumulation, "shaped like a piglet" sometimes above and sometimes below the umbilicus with pain stretching all over the abdomen and sometimes as far up as just below the heart, cold limbs, heart palpitations, and unpredictable hot and cold. It can be due to kidney qi emptiness, sexual fatigue, accumulation of cold evil, or stagnation due to *shan.*

(4) **Qi lump, chilly qi:** Moxa *Qi Hai* (CV 6).

(5) **Below the heart (epigastrium) cold as ice:** Needle and moxa *Zhong Wan* (CV 12) and *Bai Hui* (GV 20).

(6) **Phlegm stagnation becomes a lump:** Moxa 100 cones on *Fei Shu* (Bl 13), 3 cones on *Qi Men* (Liv 14).

(7) **Lower abdominal lumps or accumulations:** Moxa as many cones as the age of the patient on *Shen Shu* (Bl 23), on *Fei Shu* (Bl 13), *Da Chang Shu* (Bl 25), *Gan Shu* (Bl 18), and *Tai Chong* (Liv 3) moxa 10 cones apiece.

(8) **Abdomen inside accumulations and lumps; qi moves up and down:** Moxa 100 cones on *Zhong Ji* (CV 3). Moxa 3 cones on *Xuan Shu* (GV 5) which is located below the 13th vertebra.

Comment. This describes a condition in which the patient feels as if there is something stuck in the center of their torso and the qi must therefore move up and down the sides.

(9) **Abdominal lump:** Place one needle each in the top, center, and bottom of the lump itself, and also moxa in each place 14-21 cones. In another treatment moxa many cones on the abdominal lump point, which is located below the 11th vertebra and out 3 1/2 *cun*.

12) *HUANG DAN* (Jaundice)

(1) **Jaundice:** Needle and/or moxa *Zhi Yang* (GV 9), *Bai Lao* (extra point M-HN-30, see p. 21, section 5, #2), *San Li* (St 36), and *Zhong Wan* (CV 12).

(2) **Food jaundice:** Needle *San Li* (St 36), *Shen Men* (Ht 7), *Jian Shi* (Per 5), and *Lie Que* (Lu 7).

(3) **Alcohol (wine) jaundice:** Needle *Gong Sun* (Sp 4), *Dan Shu* (Bl 19), *Zhi Yang* (GV 9), *Wei Zhong* (Bl 40), *Wan Gu* (SI 4), *Zhong Wan* (CV 12), *Shen Men* (Ht 7), and *Xiao Chang Shu* (Bl 27).

(4) **Female taxation jaundice:** *Gong Sun* (Sp 4), *Guan Yuan* (CV 4), *Zhi Yang* (GV 9), *Shen Shu* (Bl 23), and *Ran Gu* (Ki 2); moxa all 3 cones.

(5) **36 kinds of jaundice moxa method:** First moxa *Fei Shu* (Bl 13) 3 cones, then moxa *He Gu* (LI 4) 3 cones, then moxa *Qi Hai* (CV 6) 100 cones; needle *Zhong Wan* (CV 12).

13) *NUE JI* (Malarial Disease)

Comment: The term *nue* is commonly translated into English as malaria. The term can also simply mean a disease in which the predominating symptom is alternating fever and chills. We have chosen to leave the term in Chinese *pin yin*.

(1) **Longterm *nue*, cannot recover:** Moxa *Da Zhui* (GV 14) and *Fu Liu* (Ki 7).

(2) **Warm *nue*:** Needle *Zhong Wan* (CV 12) and *Da Zhui* (GV 14).

(3) **Phlegm *nue* (with) hot and cold:** Needle *Hou Xi* (SI 3) and *He Gu* (LI 4).

(4) **Cold *nue*:** Needle *San Jian* (LI 3).

67

(5) *Nue* with much heat (fever) and little cold (chills): Needle and/or moxa *Jian Shi* (Per 5) and *San Li* (St 36).

(6) *Nue* with much cold (chills) and little heat (fever): Moxa *Fu Liu* (Ki 7) and *Da Zhui* (GV 14).

(7) Longterm *nue* which will not heal: Needle and/or moxa *Gong Sun* (Sp 4), *Nei Ting* (St 44) and *Li Dui* (St 45).

(8) Foot *tai yang nue* first cold (chills) then hot (fever) with uncontrollable sweating: Choose *Jin Men* (Bl 63).

(9) Foot *shao yang nue* with both fever and chills, heart pounding, sweat excessive: Treat *Xia Xi* (GB 43).

(10) Foot *yang ming nue* longterm cold (chills), then heat (fever); sweating profuse; patient wants to be exposed to the light and heat of a fire: Treat *Chong Yang* (St 42).

(11) Foot *tai yin nue* with sweating, tendency to vomit. After the vomiting comes exhaustion: Treat *Gong Sun* (Sp 4).

(12) Foot *shao yin nue* with extreme vomiting; one feels as if one is going to die; desire to be in a secluded place: Needle *Da Zhong* (Ki 4).

Comment: The implication here is that the disease has affected the person's spirit.

(13) Foot *jue yin nue* with lower abdomen fullness and urination inhibited: Treat *Tai Chong* (Liv 3).

(14) *Nue mu*: Needle and then moxa *Zhang Men* (Liv 13).

Comment: Literally mother of malaria, i.e., lump glomus

occurring in malarial diseases.

14) *WEN YI* (Pestilential or Acute Communicable Diseases)

(1) **Dry cholera:** Prick with a needle to draw blood at *Wei Zhong* (Bl 40) and the 10 fingers *jing* well points.

(2) **Cholera with vomiting and diarrhea that won't stop; the patient is close to death:** Moxa 1000 cones between the following points: *Tian Shu* (St 25), *Qi Hai* (CV 6), and *Zhong Wan* (CV 12).

(3) **Wringing intestine choleric condition:** Hands and feet are numb and cold, abdominal pain is unbearable. Dip hands in warm water and then sprinkle this onto the wrist and knee joints. Then pat the local area with your fingers until some black and purple spots arise. Then use a needle to prick these spots to let out the bad blood; the patient will recover instantly.

(4) **Cholera with vomiting and diarrhea (and) twisted sinews:** Needle *Zhong Wan* (CV 12), *Yin Ling* (Sp 9), *Cheng Shan* (Bl 57), *Yang Fu* (GB 38), *Tai Bai* (Sp 3), *Da Du* (Sp 2), *Zhong Feng* (Liv 4), and *Kun Lun* (Bl 60).

(5) **Cholera with dry heaves:** Moxa 7 cones on *Jian Shi* (Per 5). If it is not healed, moxa it again.

(6) **Cholera with mental confusion and depression:** Moxa 7 cones on the center of the umbilicus. Needle and moxa *Jian Li* (CV 11); needle *San Jiao Shu* (Bl 22), *He Gu* (LI 4), *Tai Chong* (Liv 3), *Guan Chong* (TH 1), and *Zhong Wan* (CV 12).

(7) **Sudden and violent outbreak of cholera:** Needle *Da Du* (Sp 2), *Kun Lun* (Bl 60), *Qi Men* (Liv 14), *Yin Ling* (Sp 9), and *Zhong Wan* (CV 12).

(8) **Fatal cholera:** If there is still body warmth moxa 7 cones on top of salt filling the umbilicus and 7 cones on top of *Da Dun* (Liv 1).

15) *DIAN XIAN* (Epilepsy)

(1) **Heart evil insanity or dementia:** Needle and/or moxa *Zan Zhu* (Bl 2), *Chi Ze* (Lu 5), *Jian Shi* (Per 5), and *Yang Xi* (LI 5).

(2) **Insanity or dementia:** Moxa 7 cones on *Qu Chi* (LI 11). Then moxa *Shao Hai* (Ht 3), *Jian Shi* (Per 5), *Yang Xi* (LI 5), *Yang Gu* (SI 5), *Da Ling* (Per 7), *He Gu* (LI 4), *Yu Ji* (Lu 10), *Wan Gu* (SI 4), *Shen Men* (Ht 7), *Ye Men* (TH 2), *Fei Shu* (Bl 13), *Xing Jian* (Liv 2), and *Jing Gu* (Bl 64). Moxa 100 cones on *Chong Yang* (St 42).

(3) **Epilepsy:** Moxa 7 cones each on *Bai Hui* (GV 20) and *Shen Men* (Ht 7); 3 cones on *Gui Yan* (Ghost Eyes, another name for *Yin Bai* [Sp 1] and *Shao Shang* [Lu 11] used together. See #2 in the pediatric section below for method); 30 cones on *Yang Xi* (LI 5) and *Jian Shi* (Per 5); 100 cones each on *Shen Men* (Ht 7), *Xin Shu* (Bl 15), *Fei Shu* (Bl 13), and 7 cones each on *Shen Mai* (Bl 62), *Chi Ze* (Lu 5), *Tai Chong* (Liv 3) and *Qu Chi* (LI 11).

(4) **Raving:** Needle and/or moxa *Tai Yuan* (Lu 9), *Yang Xi* (LI 5), *Xia Jian* (LI 8), and *Kun Lun* (Bl 60).

(5) **Manic raving:** Needle and/or moxa *Da Ling* (Per 7).

(6) **Excessive raving:** Needle and/or moxa *Bai Hui* (GV 20).

(7) **Happy smile:** Needle *Shui Gou* (GV 26), *Lie Que* (Lu 7), *Yang Xi* (LI 5), and *Da Ling* (Per 7).

Comment: This term describes a type of incessant manic giggling.

(8) **Apt to cry:** Needle *Bai Hui* (GV 20) and *Shui Gou* (GV 26).

(9) **Near death madness:** Needle *Jian Shi* (Per 5), *He Gu* (LI 4), and *Hou Xi* (SI 3).

(10) **Crazy walking or running:** Needle *Feng Fu* (GV 16) and *Yang Gu* (SI 5).

(11) **Becomes crazy:** Needle *Shao Hai* (Ht 3), *Jian Shi* (Per 5), *Shen Men* (Ht 7), *He Gu* (LI 4), *Hou Xi* (SI 3), *Fu Liu* (Ki 7), and *Si Zhu Kong* (TH 23).

(12) **Slow-witted:** Needle and/or moxa *Shen Men* (Ht 7), *Shao Shang* (Lu 11), *Yong Quan* (Ki 1), and *Xin Shu* (Bl 15).

(13) **Manic; person may tear their clothes off, run around screaming, climb on the rooftops and yell, etc.:** Needle *Shen Men* (Ht 7), *Hou Xi* (SI 3), and *Chong Yang* (St 42).

(14) **Epilepsy:** Moxa *Tian Jing* (TH 10), *Ju Que* (CV 14), *Bai Hui* (GV 20), *Shen Que* (CV 8), *Yong Quan* (Ki 1), and *Da Zhui* (GV 14); and below the 9th vertebra moxa 3 cones.

71

(15) **Ox epilepsy:** Moxa 3 cones each on *Jiu Wei* (CV 15) and *Da Zhui* (GV 14).

Comment: In China it is thought that a person having an epileptic seizure looks/behaves/sounds like a goat. Numbers 15 through 19 suggest variations on this idea. Specific symptoms for each are not available. However, it seems that the main variation would have to do with the noises that the person makes during a seizure.

(16) **Horse epilepsy:** Moxa *Pu Shen* (Bl 61), *Feng Fu* (GV 16), the center of the umbilicus, *Jin Men* (Bl 63), *Bai Hui* (GV 20), and *Shen Ting* (GV 24).

(17) **Dog epilepsy:** Moxa 3 cones on *Lao Gong* (Per 8) and *Shen Mai* (Bl 62).

(18) **Chicken epilepsy:** Moxa *Ling Dao* (Ht 4) 3 cones, needle *Jin Men* (Bl 63), and moxa 3 cones each on *Zu Lin Qi* (GB 41) and *Nei Ting* (St 44).

(19) **Swine epilepsy:** Moxa 3 cones each on *Kun Lun* (Bl 60), *Pu Shen* (Bl 61), *Yong Quan* (Ki 1), *Lao Gong* (Per 8), *Shui Gou [Ren Zhong]* (GV 26), *Bai Hui* (GV 20), *Shuai Gu* (GB 8), *Wan Gu* (SI 4), and *Nei Huai Jian* (Inner Ankle Tip M-LE-17).

(20) **The five types of epilepsy (presenting with) spittle:** Moxa 100 cones each on *Hou Xi* (SI 3), *Shen Men* (Ht 7), *Xin Shu* (Bl 15), and *Gui Yan* (Ghost Eyes, see page 75 #2). Moxa 3 cones on *Jian Shi* (Per 5).

(21) **Eyes rolled up without awareness:** Moxa *Xin Hui* (GV 22), *Ju Que* (CV 14), and *Xing Jian* (Liv 2).

16) *FU REN* (Women, i.e. Gynecology)

(1) **Irregular menstruation:** Needle and/or moxa *Qi Hai* (CV 6), *Zhong Ji* (CV 3), *Dai Mai* (GB 26), *Shen Shu* (Bl 23), and *San Yin Jiao* (Sp 6).

(2) **Excessive menstruation which does not stop:** Needle *Yin Bai* (Sp 1).

(3) **Menses flows down like water, arrives at no set time:** Moxa *Guan Yuan* (CV 4).

(4) **Dribbling down does not stop (prolonged menstruation):** Needle and/or moxa *Tai Chong* (Liv 3) and *San Yin Jiao* (Sp 6).

(5) **Blood avalanche (menorrhagia):** Consider choosing from and needling *Qi Hai* (CV 6), *Da Dun* (Liv 1), *Yin Gu* (Ki 10), *Tai Chong* (Liv 3), *Ran Gu* (Ki 2), *San Yin Jiao* (Sp 6), or *Zhong Ji* (CV 3).

(6) **No incense:** Moxa *Guan Yuan* (Cv 4) 30 cones; one might also possibly moxa *San Yin Jiao* (Sp 6), *Shi Guan* (Ki 18), *Guan Yuan* (CV 4), *Zhong Ji* (CV 3), *Shang Qiu* (Sp 5), *Yong Quan* (Ki 1), and *Zhu Bin* (Ki 9).

Comment: No incense is a polite way of describing infertility. When a woman is pregnant, her family and friends will offer incense at the local temple, requesting her and the child's protection and health.

(7) **Slippery fetus (habitual abortion):** Moxa 2 *cun* to the left and right of *Guan Yuan* (CV 4) 50 cones, possibly moxa 3 *cun* to the left and right of *Zhong Ji* (CV 3).

73

(8) **Difficult birth destroys, pass down dead fetus:** Tonify *Tai Chong* (Liv 3); tonify *He Gu* (LI 4); disperse *San Yin Jiao* (Sp 6).

(9) **Transverse delivery, hand exits ahead:** Moxa the tip of the small toe 3 cones.

(10) **Afterbirth does not descend:** Needle *San Yin Jiao* (Sp 6), *Zhong Ji* (CV 3), *Zhao Hai* (Ki 6), *Nei Guan* (Per 6), and *Kun Lun* (Bl 60).

(11) **Postpartum anemic fainting and dizziness:** Needle *San Li* (St 36), *San Yin Jiao* (Sp 6), *Zhi Gou* (TH 6), *Shen Men* (Ht 7), and *Nei Guan* (Per 6).

(12) **Red and white vaginal discharge:** Moxa *Qu Gu* (CV 2) 7 cones and *Tai Chong* (Liv 3), *Nei Guan* (Per 6), *Fu Liu* (Ki 7), and *Tian Shu* (St 25) 100 cones.

(13) ***Gan xue lao* (a type of consumptive disease in women characterized by menostasis, recurrent low fever, and general debility):** Needle and/or moxa *Qu Chi* (LI 11), *Zhi Gou* (TH 6), *San Li* (St 36), and *San Yin Jiao* (Sp 6).

(14) **Postpartum exhaustion:** Needle and/or moxa *Bai Lao* (M-HN-30) *Shen Shu* (Bl 23), *Feng Men* (Bl 12), *Zhong Ji* (CV 3), *Qi Hai* (CV 6), and *San Yin Jiao* (Sp 6).

(15) **Agalactia:** Moxa *Shan Zhong* (CV 17) and tonify *Shao Ze* (SI 1).

(16) **Postpartum blood lump pain:** Needle *Qu Quan* (Liv 8), *Fu Liu* (Ki 7), *San Li* (St 36), *Qi Hai* (CV 6), and *Nei Guan* (Per 6).

17) *XIAO ER KE* (Pediatrics)

(1) **Navel wind, i.e. umbilical tetanus with lockjaw:** Needle *Ran Gu* (Ki 2) 3 *fen,* moxa 3 cones.

Comment: Tetanus infection of the umbilicus often happened in times past due to unclean surgical instruments and lack of knowledge about hygiene.

(2) **Fright epilepsy, i.e. convulsions:** Moxa *Gui Yan,* the Ghost Eyes points (bind the thumbs and big toes of the hands and feet together side by side and moxa the hollow under the nails, i.e., *Shao Shang* [Lu 11] and *Yin Bai* [Sp 1]).

(3) **Fright wind, i.e. convulsions:** Needle *Wan Gu* (SI 4).

(4) **Anal prolapse:** Moxa *Bai Hui* (GV 20) 7 cones and *Chang Qiang* (GV 1) 3 cones.

(5) **Fright wind, convulsions, critical and recalcitrant to treatment:** Moxa beneath both nipples above the dark flesh 3 cones.

(6) **Diarrhea, dysentery:** Moxa *Shen Que* (CV 8).

(7) **Cold dysentery:** Moxa 2 *cun* beneath the navel.

(8) **Vomiting milk:** Moxa 1 *cun,* 6 *fen* below *Shan Zhong* (CV 17) and also *Zhong Ting* (CV 16) 5 cones.

(9) **Frothy vomit and dead faint:** Moxa *Ju Que* (CV 14) 7 cones and *Zhong Wan* (CV 12) 50 cones.

(10) **Opistothonis (seen in tetanus during convulsions):** Moxa

Bai Hui (GV 20) 7 cones and *Tian Tu* (CV 22) 3 cones.

(11) **Night crying:** Moxa *Bai Hui* (GV 20) 3 cones.

(12) **Umbilical swelling:** Moxa 3, possibly as many as 7 cones above the backbone opposite the umbilicus.

(13) **Erosion of the mouth and gums with bad breath:** Moxa *Lao Gong* (Per 8) 1 cone.

(14) **Unilateral swelling and prolapse of the kidney:** Moxa *Guan Yuan* (CV 4) 3 cones and *Da Dun* (Liv 1) 7 cones.

(15) **Sores on one side of the body:** Needle *Qu Chi* (LI 11), *He Gu* (LI 4), *San Li* (St 36), *Jue Gu* (GB 39), and *Xi Yan* (St 35).

(16) **Bedwetting:** *Qi Hai* (CV 6) moxa 100 cones, *Da Dun* (Liv 1) 3 cones.

(17) **Emaciation, food not transforming:** Moxa *Wei Shu* (Bl 21) and *Chang Gu* (Long Valley, 2 *cun* on either side of the umbilicus) 7 cones.

18) *YANG ZHONG* (Ulcerous Sores and Swellings)

(1) **Carbuncle, deep-rooted ulcer, toxic swelling:** Moxa above the initial place the swelling appeared 7 cones; if it has already broken through, possible transformation into Toxins may be perilous, therefore urgently moxa *Qi Zhu Ma* (Ride the Bamboo Horse point (this point is difficult to locate; approximately 1/2 *cun* lateral to the process of T 10; must be found by palpation).

(2) **Furunculous swelling on the face:** Needle and/or moxa *He Gu* (LI 4), *Zu San Li* (St 36), and *Shen Men* (Ht 7).

(3) **Furunculous swelling on the hand:** Moxa *Qu Chi* (LI 11).

(4) **Furunculous swelling on the back:** Needle and/or moxa *Jian Jing* (GB 21), *San Li* (St 36), *Wei Zhong* (Bl 40), *Lin Qi* (GB 41), *Xing Jian* (Liv 2), *Tong Li* (Ht 6), *Shao Hai* (Ht 3), and *Tai Chong* (Liv 3) while simultaneously moxaing *Qi Zhu Ma* point.

(5) **Carbuncle or deep-rooted ulcer erupting on the back which initially is not painful:** Apply a slice of garlic over the site and crown with artemesia moxa. If there is no carbuncle, the moxa will hurt. If there is pain, moxa until the pain stops. **Bone ulcer:** Employ moxa 1 *cun* behind *Jian Shi* (Per 5) as many cones as the patient's years of age.

(6) **Scabious sores:** Needle *Fei Shu* (Bl 13), *Shen Men* (Ht 7), *Da Ling* (Per 7), and *Qu Chi* (LI 11).

(7) **Sabre and bead goitre (lymphadenitis scrofulosa of the neck and axilla):** Moxa *Jue Gu* (GB 39) and *Shen Men* (Ht 7).

(8) **Hot wind addiction rash (due to alcoholism):** Needle *Qu Chi* (LI 11), *Qu Ze* (Per 3), *He Gu* (LI 4), *Lie Que* (Lu 7), *Fei Shu* (Bl 13), *Yu Ji* (Lu 10), *Shen Men* (Ht 7), and *Nei Guan* (Per 6).

(9) **Skin wind itch and rash:** Moxa *Qu Chi* (LI 11) 200 cones, and *Shen Men* (Ht 7) and *He Gu* (LI 4) 37 cones.

(10) **Scrofula:** Moxa *Bai Lao* (M-HN-30) 37-100 cones and

the tip of the elbow 100 cones. First pierce with a needle the scrofulous lumps right through their center. Use moxa made from artemesia mixed with realgar powder.

(11) **Gall or goitre lump or tumor:** Treat goitre by moxaing *Tian Tu* (CV 22) 37 cones. Also moxa *Jian Yu* (LI 5). For a man, moxa the left point 18 cones and the right 17 cones. For a woman, moxa the right 18 cones and the left 17 cones.

(12) **Big wind sore (leprosy):** Using a 3-edged needle, inspect the flesh looking for purple reaching up to *Wei Zhong* (Bl 40). Bleed the purple vein. However, nowadays, it is not ok to bleed too much for fear of decreasing the true qi.

(13) ***Gan lou*, lymphadenitis or fistula associated with pediatric malnutrition:** If there are chronic oozing sores, moxa 1 *cun* above the medial malleolus 3 cones. If there are sores on the upper body, as a rule moxa *Jian Jing* (GB 21) and *Jiu Wei* (CV 15). For cold, copious leakage existing between the leg and foot, one should use the aconite and moxa method or the sulfur and moxa method. This is even if initially the sore was due to accumulated heat pouring downward, since chronic conditions typically become cold. For longterm sores which leak continiously pusy water, one should also moxa.

Index

abdomen hard 63
abdominal distention 62, 63
abdominal lumps 66
abdominal pain 13, 30, 32, 33, 42,
53, 58, 69
    at the navel 32
    indigestion 32
    lancinating 32
    lower 33
    with hardness 63
abortion, habitual 73
accumulation pain 32
acid regurgitation 58
afterbirth won't descend 74
agalactia 32, 74
anal prolapse 47, 48, 75
ankle 38, 39
    pain 37
    sore 39
anus 47, 48
appetite reduced 58
apt to cry 71
arms 34-36
    cannot bend 35
    cannot lift 35
    chilly pain 35
    numbness 35
    red and swollen 35
    sore and contracted 36
arthritis 51
asthma 7, 61
    moxa method 61
axilla 36, 77
    swollen 36

backache 27

bedwetting 76
ben tun 65
beng lou 10, 47
bi patterns 50, 51
biliary ascariasis 11
birthing difficult 74
black circles around eye 20
bleeding 5, 6, 73
    after defecation 48
    from lower body 5
    nose 5
    uterine 10
    with cough 5
    with vomit 5
    with feces 5, 48, 51
blindness 19
    night blindness 19
    sudden 19
blood in the feces 5, 48, 51
body hot 54, 56, 59
bone *bi* 50
bone pain 42
bones soft, no power 42
borborygmus 33
brain pain 17
breast 28, 31, 32
    swollen 32
    mastitis 32
    agalactia 32
    hypergalactia 31
    pain 32

carbuncle 76, 77
cataract 20
chaotic qi 3
cheeks swollen 17

chest cold 30
chest fullness 30
chest pain 28, 30, 54
        obstruction 29
chest quivering 30
chest stuffy 29
cholera 69, 70
clear-eyed blindness 19
cold injury 8, 29, 51-55, 60
consumptive diseases 59, 74
consumptive heat 56
constipation (stools stopped up)
14
        due to cold injury 54
        in post-partum women
        14
convulsions 75
corneal opacity 18, 20
cough 56, 59-61
        due to cold injury 60
        counterflow 60
        difficulty sleeping 59, 60
        longterm 59
        with pain in flanks 61
        with pain in lumbar 61
        with phlegm 59
        with wheezing 59, 60
coughing blood 5
crazy 71
crying 71

damp 56
deafness 20, 21
        sudden 21
        hard of hearing 21
dementia 70
diabetic polydipsia 22
diaphragm blockage 58
diarrhea 13, 33, 47, 48, 69, 75
        explosive 47
dizziness 15-17, 74
dreams 1, 6

dribbling 11, 12, 45, 73
dry heaves 41, 62, 69
dry mouth 57
duck stools (watery) 32
dullness, stupidity 4
dysentery 13, 14, 48, 75
dyspnea 59, 60

ear 20
        pus, water flows from
        ear   21
edema 9, 64
        any type 64
        chest, abdomen 64
        eyes 64
        facial 64
        four limbs 64
        superficial 64
elbow contraction, pain 34
emaciation 76
empty fatigue 1, 59
empty taxation 59
unurouo 13
epilepsy 4, 50, 70-72, 75
essence 1, 3
eyeball pain 17
eyelashes fall out 19
eyelids 18
eyes 17-19
        itch 19
        red 17
        roll back in head 19, 72
        swollen 17

face itchy 17
face puffy 64
face swollen 17
fear of cold 15
fever due to cold injury 52, 54
fingers
        cannot bend 35

painful 34
rigid 34, 35
spastic 34
fistula 78
five consumptive diseases 59
flaccid tongue 8, 24
flank pain 30, 31, 54
flank and chest distended 31
floating beam 65
food stagnation 32
food won't descend 58
foot (feet)
    cold and hot 38
    cold like ice 38, 39, 56
    emaciated 37
    feeble/weak 39
    pain 38, 39
    foot qi 40
    senseless 38
    sinew twisted 39
    sore 39
    swollen 39
    weak 37
forearm cold 34
forearm pain 34
frequent urination 12, 20, 44
fright palpitations 6
fright wind (convulsions) 75
furunculous swelling 77

gan lou 78
gan xue lao 74
goitre 77, 78

habitual abortion 73
hands
    cannot bend 35
    chilly pain 35
    heat in palms 35
    numb 34, 35
    pain 34

red 35
rigid 34
shaking 34
spastic 34
swollen 35
without strength 35
head wind 16
headache 15-17, 51-53
    bilateral 17
    due to cold injury 53
    entire head 16
    kidney inversion 16
    migraine 15
    one-sided 17
heart 3, 4, 27-30, 33, 35, 57, 58, 63, 65, 66, 68, 70
heart and chest pain 30
heart pain 27-29, 33
    abrupt 28
    blood heart pain 29
    due to obstruction 28
    due to worms 28
    extending to the back 28
    subclavicular fossa area 29
heart stagnation 65
heart vexation 57
heartburn 28
heaviness 6, 14
hemafecia 4, 48, 51
hemiplegia 49
hemorrhoid 47, 48
    longterm 48
    moxa method 48
    with bleeding 48
hernia 33, 42, 46, 47
hunger 58
hydrocele 44
hypergalactia (jealous milk) 31
hysteric raving 4

incontinent 48
indifference to food 57
indigestion 32
infertility (no incense) 73
injury due to cold 51-56
insanity 70
insomnia 6
intercostal pain 30
intestinal wind 48
intestinal wringing 69
intoxication 17
inversion of qi 2
inverted cup 65
inverted qi 2, 7, 65

jaundice 66, 67
jing 1, 9, 10, 18, 19, 26-30, 35, 36,
43, 47, 50, 53, 55, 56, 61, 62,
69-71, 77, 78
joints all sore 51

knee 37
        bent, cannot relax 41
        inside painful 37
        outside painful 37
        painful 37
        red 39
        swollen 37

lack of will 4
laryngeal pain 25
leg collapses 37
leg flaccid 36
leg/knee spasm 36
leg
        pain 36
        paralysis 38
        senseless 38
        slack 39
        sore 38

spasm 39
swollen 39
legs feel like ice 37
leprosy 78
leukorrhea 1, 10, 12
limbs swollen 64
limbs cold 13
        inversion chill 41, 55
lin 11, 20, 29, 32, 36, 37, 45, 52,
54, 56, 72, 77
        stone *lin* 11
        qi *lin* 11, 45
        blood *lin* 11
lip swollen 23
lips dry 22, 23
lockjaw 50, 75
loose stools 13
loss of appetite 57, 58
loss of consciousness 7, 54
loss of sperm 2
loss of voice 7
lower abdominal lumps 66
lumbar pain 33, 34
        cannot stand up straight
           33
        kidney emptiness 33
        due to sprain 33
        with stiffness 33
        as if sitting in water 34
        difficult to move 34
lump glomus (*nue mu*) 68
lung lump 65
lymphadenitis 26, 77, 78

malaria 67, 68
mania 4, 54
mastitis 32
memory impaired 4
menopause 10
menorrhagia 10, 73
menostasis 74
menses 73

menstruation 9, 10, 73
       excessive 73
       irregular 73
migraine 15
mouth deviated 49
mouth erosion 76
mouth sores 22
muteness 7

nasal polyps 22
navel wind (umbilical tetanus) 75
neck pain 26
night crying 76
night sweat 8, 59
no pulse 41, 55
nose
       bleed 5
       runny 21
       stuffed 21
       nasal polyps 22
       prolonged mucous 22
nue 67, 68
numbness of the hand 35

opisthotonis 16, 26, 50, 55

paralysis
       leg 38
       mouth 50
       one-sided 49
parasites 11, 28
pediatric malnutrition 78
penis pain 44
pharynx obstructed 25
phlegm fluid 9
phlegm stagnation 66
postpartum anemic fainting 74
postpartum exhaustion 74
postpartum blood lump pain 74
prolapse 43, 76

       of kidney 76
ptergium 18
pulses gone 40, 55

qi counterflow 60
qi lump 66

raving 4, 70, 71
red urine 45
reluctance to speak 57
retention of urine 11
rheumatic arthritis 51
rib pain 31
ribs and spine pulled together 31
running piggy 65
runny nose 21, 22

saliva drips down 24
scabious sores 77
scrofula 77
scrofulous sores 40
scrotal pain 46
shan 5, 14, 17, 25, 30, 38, 39, 41-44, 46-48, 55, 60-62, 65, 69, 74, 75
       cold *shan* 42
       fetal *shan* 43
       foxy *shan* 43
       lump pain 44
       miscellaneous 46
       moxa method 46
       sudden *shan* 44
       testicular *shan* 44
       ulcerous *shan* 43, 76
       water ulcer 43
       with prolapse 43
       woman's *shan* 43
       yin *shan* 44
shen (spirit) 3
shin cold 38

shin pain 36, 37
sighing 2
sinew *bi* 51
sinew pattern due to liver heat 41
sinews contracted 41, 42
sinews twisted and painful 42
skin 40

       feels like worms crawling on 40

       bi 51

       wind itch 77

       rash 77

sleepiness 6
slippery fetus 12, 73
slow-witted 71
small intestine qi (hernia) 46
somnolence 57
spasm of the leg 39
spermatorrhea 1, 45
spinal column stiff 26
spine stiff 42
steaming bone 56, 59
stomach heat 57
stomach reflux 61
stomach upset 58
stomach weakness 57
stools stopped up 14
stuffy chest 29
stuffy flanks 30
stupidity 4
subaxillary swelling 36
subclavicular fossa pain 29
sublingual swelling 8
superciliary ridge pain 17
superficial edema 64
sweating 8, 52, 53, 68

       too little 8

       too much 8, 53

       night 8

       lack of 8, 52

swollen feet 39
swollen legs 39

tearing (in the wind) 19
teeth, dry 56
tenesmus 14
tendency to cry 71
terrified 6
testicle enlarged, rigid 46
testicle painful 46
testicles enter abdomen 44
testicular swelling 33, 43, 44
tetanus 75
thief (night) sweating 8
thigh pain 37
thigh pivot pain 38
thirst 13, 22, 57
throat constricted as if a fish bone were caught inside 25
throat swollen 25
throat obstruction 7, 24, 25
throat pain 25
thoracic glomus 29
tinnitus 20
toes painful 37
tongue

       flaccid 24

       stiff 24

tongue swollen 23
tonsilitis (milky moth) 25
tooth pain 16, 24
transverse delivery 74

ulcer, watery 43
umbilical swelling 76
umbilical tetanus 75
unable to lie down 6
urethra pain 12
urination 11-13

       frequent 12

       blocked 12, 54

       turbid 12, 45

       slippery 12

       with blood 45

urine dark 45

urine not free flowing 54
urine red 45
uterine bleeding 10, 75
uterus retroversion 45

vaginal discharge 10, 11, 74
vertigo 15
violent mania 4
vitiligo 40
vomiting 5, 9, 13, 52, 58, 59, 61,
62, 68, 69, 75
vomiting bitter water 61
vomiting blood 5

warts 40
water swelling 63, 64
water ulcer 43
watery stools 32
wet dreams 1
wheezing 59, 60
white turbidity (urine) 45
wind stroke 49, 50
            omens of 50
wrist pain 36
wooden kidney 46

yawning 2
yin toxins 54

OTHER BOOKS ON CHINESE MEDICINE
AVAILABLE FROM
BLUE POPPY PRESS

1775 Linden Ave
Boulder, CO 80304
PH. 303\442-0796 FAX 303\447-0740

PMS: Its Cause, Diagnosis & Treatment According to Traditional Chinese Medicine by Bob Flaws ISBN 0-936185-22-8 $14.95

SOMETHING OLD, SOMETHING NEW; Essays on the TCM Description of Western Herbs, Pharmaceuticals, Vitamins & Minerals by Bob Flaws ISBN 0-936185-21-X $19.95

SCATOLOGY & THE GATE OF LIFE: The Role of the Large Intestine in Immunity, An Integrated Chinese-Western Approach by Bob Flaws ISBN 0-936185-20-1 $12.95

SECOND SPRING: A Guide To Healthy Menopause Through Traditional Chinese Medicine by Honora Lee Wolfe ISBN 0-936185-18-X $14.95

MIGRAINES & TRADITIONAL CHINESE MEDICINE: A Layperson's Guide by Bob Flaws ISBN 0-936185-15-5 $11.95

STICKING TO THE POINT: A Rational Methodology for the Step by Step Formulation & Administration of an Acupuncture Treatment by Bob Flaws ISBN 0-936185-17-1 $14.95

ENDOMETRIOSIS & INFERTILITY AND TRADITIONAL CHINESE MEDICINE: A Laywoman's Guide by Bob Flaws ISBN 0-936185-14-7 $9.95

CLASSICAL MOXIBUSTION SKILLS IN CONTEMPORARY CLINICAL PRACTICE by Sung Baek ISBN 0-936185-16-3 $10.95

THE BREAST CONNECTION: A Laywoman's Guide to the Treatment of Breast Disease by Chinese Medicine by Honora Lee Wolfe ISBN 0-936185-13-9 $8.95

NINE OUNCES: A Nine Part Program For The Prevention of AIDS in HIV Positive Persons by Bob Flaws ISBN 0-936185-12-0 $9.95

THE TREATMENT OF
CANCER BY INTEGRATED
CHINESE-WESTERN
MEDICINE by Zhang Dai-
zhao, trans. by Zhang Ting-liang
& Bob Flaws, ISBN 0-936185-
11-2 $16.95

BLUE POPPY ESSAYS: 1988
**Translations and
Ruminations on Chinese
Medicine** by Flaws, Chace et al,
ISBN 0-936185-10-4 $18.95

A HANDBOOK OF
TRADITIONAL CHINESE
DERMATOLOGY by Liang
Jian-hui, trans. by Zhang Ting-
liang & Bob Flaws, ISBN 0-
936185-07-4 $14.95

SECRET SHAOLIN
FORMULAE FOR THE
TREATMENT OF
EXTERNAL INJURY by
Patriarch De Chan, trans. by
Zhang Ting-liang & Bob Flaws,
ISBN 0-936185-08-2 $13.95

A HANDBOOK OF
TRADITIONAL CHINESE
GYNECOLOGY by Zhejiang
College of TCM, trans. by
Zhang Ting-liang, ISBN 0-
936185-06-6 (2nd edit.) $21.95

FREE & EASY: Traditional
Chinese Gynecology for
American Women 2nd Edition,
by Bob Flaws, ISBN 0-936185-
05-8 $15.95

PRINCE WEN HUI'S
COOK: Chinese Dietary
Therapy by Bob Flaws &
Honora Lee Wolfe, ISBN 0-
912111-05-4, $12.95 (Published
by Paradigm Press, Brookline,
MA)

TURTLE TAIL & OTHER
TENDER MERCIES:
**Traditional Chinese
Pediatrics** by Bob Flaws ISBN
0-936185-00-7 $14.95

THE DAO OF INCREASING
LONGEVITY AND
CONSERVING ONE'S LIFE
by Anna Lin & Bob Flaws,
ISBN 0-936185-24-4 $16.95

FIRE IN THE VALLEY: The
**TCM Diagnosis and
Treatment of Vaginal
Diseases** by Bob Flaws
ISBN 0-936185-25-2 $16.95

HIGHLIGHTS OF ANCIENT
ACUPUNCTURE
PRESCRIPTIONS trans. by
Honora Lee Wolfe & Rose
Crescenz ISBN 0-936185-23-6
$14.95